Virtue Ethics

Blackwell Readings in Philosophy
Series Editor: Steven M. Cahn

Blackwell Readings in Philosophy are concise, chronologically arranged collections of primary readings from classical and contemporary sources. They represent core positions and important developments with respect to key philosophical concepts. Edited and introduced by leading philosophers, these volumes provide valuable resources for teachers and students of philosophy, and for all those interested in gaining a solid understanding of central topics in philosophy.

Virtue Ethics

Edited by

Stephen Darwall

Blackwell
Publishing

350 Main Street, Malden, MA 02148-5018, USA
108 Cowley Road, Oxford OX4 1JF, UK
550 Swanston Street, Carlton, Victoria 3053, Australia
Kurfürstendamm 57, 10707 Berlin, Germany

First published 2003 by Blackwell Publishers Ltd, a Blackwell Publishing
company

Library of Congress Cataloging-in-Publication Data

Virtue ethics / edited by Stephen Darwall.
p. cm. – (Blackwell readings in philosophy; 10)
Includes bibliographical references and index.
ISBN 0-631-23113-7 (alk. paper) – ISBN 0-631-23114-5 (pbk. : alk. paper)
1. Virtue. 2. Ethics. I. Darwall, Stephen L., 1946– II. Series.

BJ1531 .V57 2002
179'9 – dc21   2002066422

A catalogue record for this title is available from the British Library.

Set in 10/12½ Palatino
by SNP Best-set Typesetter Ltd., Hong Kong
Printed and bound in the United Kingdom
by MPG Books, Bodmin, Cornwall

For further information on
Blackwell Publishing, visit our website:
http://www.blackwellpublishing.com

Contents

Acknowledgments

I am indebted to Steven Cahn for initially suggesting the idea of this anthology, to Jeff Dean for patiently shepherding me through the production process, to Blackwell's anonymous referees for very helpful comments, to Anthony Grahame for expert copy-editing, and to Sue London for yeoman work in copying.

The editor and publisher gratefully acknowledge the following for permission to reproduce copyright material:

Chapter 1: reprinted by permission of Oxford University Press from Aristotle, *The Nicomachean Ethics*, translated with an introduction by Davis Ross, revised by J. L. Ackrill and J. O. Urmson (Oxford World's Classics, 1998);

Chapter 2: reprinted by permission of Orion Publishing Group Ltd from Francis Hutcheson, *An Inquiry into the Original of Our Idea of Virtue* (1994);

Chapter 3: reprinted by permission of Oxford University Press from David Hume, *Enquiries Concerning Human Understanding and the Principles of Morals*, edited by L. A. Selby-Bigge, revised by P. H. Nidditch (3rd edition, 1975);

Chapter 4: Philippa Foot, "Virtues and Vices" from *Virtues and Vices* (1978). Reprinted by permission of the author;

Chapter 5: John McDowell, "Virtue and Reason," *The Monist* (July 1979). Copyright © The Monist, Peru, Illinois 61354. Reprinted by permission.

Chapter 6: Alasdair MacIntyre, "The Nature of the Virtues" from *After Virtue* (1985). Reprinted by permission of University of Notre Dame Press and Duckworth Ltd;

Chapter 7: Annette Baier, "What do women want in moral theory?" from *Noûs* 19 (1985). Reprinted by permission of Blackwell Publishing.

Chapter 8: reprinted by permission of Oxford University Press from Rosalind Hursthouse, *How Should One Live?: Essays on the Virtues*, edited by Roger Crisp (1996).

Chapter 9: Michael Slote, "Agent-Based Virtue Ethics" from *Midwest Studies in Philosophy* 20 (1995). Reprinted by permission of the journal.

Chapter 10: Gary Watson, "The Primacy of Character" from *Identity, Character, and Morality*, edited by Owen Flanagan and Amelie Rorty (1990). Reproduced by permission of MIT Press.

The publisher apologizes for any errors or omissions in the above list and would be grateful if notified of any corrections that should be incorporated in future reprints or editions of this book.

Introduction

Consequentialism, contractarianism/contractualism, and deontology are all *moral* theories.[1] They concern distinctive moral notions of obligation, concern and respect and, ultimately, questions of right conduct: what we can be held morally accountable for *doing*. The approach called *virtue ethics* is orthogonal to these theories in both respects. First, virtue is concerned primarily with character rather than conduct – with how we should *be* rather than what we should *do*. And second, a virtue ethics can be advanced, not as a moral theory at all, but as an account of other, ethically deep aspects of human life that are, it is sometimes argued, potential rivals to and perhaps replacements for morality and its distinctive forms.

The conception of a set of universal and finally authoritative norms or laws by which all moral agents are categorically *obligated* is far from the only form that ethical reflection can take.[2] The modern idea of morality derives from a distinctive historical tradition, the Judaeo-Christian-Islamic idea of divinely ordained law, to which it is a secular successor. Some philosophers have argued that this conception of morality is seriously defective in various ways and that our ethical reflections might more profitably take other forms. Several who have made this argument have looked to Aristotle's *Nicomachean Ethics* for a more promising ethical conception.[3] For Aristotle, the fundamental question is not, as for Mill, Hobbes, or Kant, What is the fundamental principle of moral right or duty and how might this be defended philosophically? Aristotle asks, rather, What is the goal of human life? What kind of life is best for human beings?

Nonmoral Virtue Ethics

Aristotle provides a distinctive example – a paradigm, really – of a *non-moral virtue ethics*. ("Nonmoral," again, because, although his translators frequently use "moral virtue" to signal that he means excellences of character concerned with choice, Aristotle does not relate these to any conception of a moral law under which all are accountable as equals.) Virtues, for Aristotle, are dispositions to choose what is fine or noble (*kalon*) for its own sake, and to avoid what is base. The operative notion is what Nietzsche called a "rank-ordering" *ideal* with respect to which one can be better or worse, not a norm or law that one complies with or violates. For Aristotle, the operative ethical emotions are shame, esteem, pride and disdain or contempt, not guilt, respect, self-respect, and moral indignation.

Virtues are excellences, traits, that is, that make something an excellent instance of its kind. In this way, Aristotle's theory is a kind of *perfectionism*. It is a virtue in a knife, for example, that it have a sharp edge so that it can cut well. In general, we reckon which traits are excellences (excellent-making) in relation to a thing's function (*ergon*) or characteristic activity.[4] As Aristotle believes that the characteristic activity of human beings is action (*praxis*) that expresses a distinctively human form of choice, namely, of actions valued in themselves as noble or fine (*kalon*), he concludes that the virtues are traits of character, that is, settled dispositions to choose certain actions and avoid others as intrinsically noble or base. We might put his point by saying that human excellences are states of character concerned with choices that are themselves guided by an ideal of human excellence.

In general, any such (nonmoral) human ideal can be a nonmoral virtue ethics. Although it might involve a teleological or perfectionist view of human nature, like Aristotle's (according to which there is something human beings are inherently *for* or *to be*), it need not. A nonmoral virtue ethics may be advanced simply as a normative view about which traits in human beings are worthy of esteem (or disdain).

Moral Virtue Ethics

Analogously, a *moral virtue ethics* is a theory of what is worthy of distinctively *moral* esteem, that is, worthy of esteem *in a moral agent*. The best example of such a view is the eighteenth-century Scottish philosopher

Francis Hutcheson. Hutcheson argued that the basic moral phenomenon is a distinctively moral esteem for benevolence, the desire to benefit others and make them happy. Moral esteem, he held, is not primarily for any outcome, but for a motive or trait of character, namely, the desire to produce good outcomes for human beings and other sentient beings.

Virtue and Conduct

How, then, do virtue ethics bear on what to do? First, nonmoral virtue ethics remind us that questions of right and wrong are far from the only, or perhaps even the most important, ethical questions we can ask, even about what to do. Thus, it might be that failing to do significantly more to relieve world hunger, although famine relief is not morally obligatory, nonetheless manifests vices of complacency and self-satisfaction. Or, for another example, even if the environment cannot be wronged or unjustly treated, clear-cutting may still manifest an inappropriate attitude towards the environment or unlovely traits that are at odds with living a fully satisfying human life.

Second, in considering what to do, it can be helpful to ask what a virtuous person, or someone with a specific virtue (say, generosity), would do. This may simply be a useful heuristic, but it may also reflect the Aristotelian view that there is no way of formulating ethical insight that can be grasped and applied by someone who lacks the wisdom or "sense" of the virtuous person. As Louis Armstrong is reputed to have said about jazz, "If you have to ask, you'll never know."

Third, virtue ethicists sometimes put forward conceptions of virtue, not simply as guides to appropriate (or morally right) action, but as accounts of what *makes* an action appropriate or morally right. Thus, it can be held that an action is the right or appropriate thing to do in some case or circumstance just in case it is what the virtuous person would (characteristically) do in that circumstance.[5] Such a view might depart from the letter of Aristotle's position, since he identified virtues as settled dispositions to choose specific actions for their own sake (as noble). This would seem to make which traits are virtuous depend on which actions are noble, not vice versa. Nevertheless, since it would hold that no access to the appropriateness of action is possible save through the wisdom or conduct of a virtuous person, such a view would remain quite close to Aristotle's in fundamental spirit. What is common to any virtue ethics is the idea that guidance on controversial questions of case ethics can be gained only by looking to the virtues or the virtuous person as a model.

The readings that follow fall into three main categories: classical sources, contemporary work within virtue theory, and contemporary discussion of character and virtue. In the first category are included the classical example of a nonmoral virtue theory (Aristotle's) as well as a classical example of a moral virtue theory (Francis Hutcheson's) and Hume's esteem-based virtue theory, which problematizes the moral/nonmoral distinction. Contemporary virtue theory is represented by Philippa Foot, John McDowell, Alasdair MacIntyre, Annette Baier, Rosalind Hursthouse, and Michael Slote. Finally, there is a contemporary discussion of virtue by Gary Watson.

Notes

1 For classical and contemporary readings on these theories, see the following Blackwell anthologies (detailed on p. ii): *Consequentialism, Contractarianism/ Contractualism*, and *Deontology*.

2 G. E. M. Anscombe argued that since, as she claimed, the conception of morality is unintelligible without the idea of divine sanction, it cannot be secularized ("Modern Moral Philosophy"). Alasdair MacIntyre also advanced a very influential critique of orthodox moral philosophy (*After Virtue* [Notre Dame, IN: University of Notre Dame Press, 1981]). Bernard Williams also influentially criticized the idea of morality and its distinctive form of obligation (*Ethics and the Limits of Philosophy* [Cambridge, MA: Harvard University Press, 1985]). These writers all pointed toward Aristotle as an alternative model. See also Michael Slote, *From Morality to Virtue* (New York: Oxford University Press, 1992).

3 For a discussion of Aristotle's ethics, see my *Philosophical Ethics* (Boulder, CO: Westview Press, 1998).

4 See pp. 8–9 of this volume.

5 For an example of such a view, see Rosalind Hursthouse, *On Virtue Ethics* (Oxford: Oxford University Press, 1999).

Part I

Classical Sources

1

From *The Nicomachean Ethics*

Aristotle

Book I, 7–8

*The good must be something final and self-sufficient. Definition of happiness
reached by considering the characteristic function of man*

7.   Let us again return to the good we are seeking, and ask what it can
be. It seems different in different actions and arts; it is different in
medicine, in strategy, and in the other arts likewise. What then is the good
of each? Surely that for whose sake everything else is done. In medicine
this is health, in strategy victory, in architecture a house, in any other
sphere something else, and in every action and pursuit the end; for it is
for the sake of this that all men do whatever else they do. Therefore, if
there is an end for all that we do, this will be the good achievable by
action, and if there are more than one, these will be the goods achievable
by action.

So the argument has by a different course reached the same point; but
we must try to state this even more clearly. Since there are evidently more
than one end, and we choose some of these (e.g. wealth, flutes,[1] and in
general instruments) for the sake of something else, clearly not all ends
are final ends; but the chief good is evidently something final. Therefore,
if there is only one final end, this will be what we are seeking, and if there
are more than one, the most final of these will be what we are seeking.
Now we call that which is in itself worthy of pursuit more final than that
which is worthy of pursuit for the sake of something else, and that which
is never desirable for the sake of something else more final than the things

Aristotle, *The Nicomachean Ethics*, W. D. Ross, trans. (Oxford: Oxford University
Press, 1998), pp. 11–17, 28–47, 63–78, 137–58.

that are desirable both in themselves and for the sake of that other thing, and therefore we call final without qualification that which is always desirable in itself and never for the sake of something else.

Now such a thing happiness, above all else, is held to be; for this we choose always for itself and never for the sake of something else, but honour, pleasure, reason, and every virtue we choose indeed for themselves (for if nothing resulted from them we should still choose each of them), but we choose them also for the sake of happiness, judging that through them we shall be happy. Happiness, on the other hand, no one chooses for the sake of these, nor, in general, for anything other than itself.

From the point of view of self-sufficiency the same result seems to follow; for the final good is thought to be self-sufficient. Now by self-sufficient we do not mean that which is sufficient for a man by himself, for one who lives a solitary life, but also for parents, children, wife, and in general for his friends and fellow citizens, since man is born for citizenship. But some limit must be set to this; for if we extend our requirement to ancestors and descendants and friends' friends we are in for an infinite series. Let us examine this question, however, on another occasion;[2] the self-sufficient we now define as that which when isolated makes life desirable and lacking in nothing; and such we think happiness to be; and further we think it most desirable of all things, not a thing counted as one good thing among others – if it were so counted it would clearly be made more desirable by the addition of even the least of goods; for that which is added becomes an excess of goods, and of goods the greater is always more desirable. Happiness, then, is something final and self-sufficient, and is the end of action.

Presumably, however, to say that happiness is the chief good seems a platitude, and a clearer account of what it is is still desired. This might perhaps be given, if we could first ascertain the function of man. For just as for a flute-player, a sculptor, or any artist, and, in general, for all things that have a function or activity, the good and the 'well' is thought to reside in the function, so would it seem to be for man, if he has a function. Have the carpenter, then, and the tanner certain functions or activities, and has man none? Is he born without a function? Or as eye, hand, foot, and in general each of the parts evidently has a function, may one lay it down that man similarly has a function apart from all these? What then can this be? Life seems to belong even to plants, but we are seeking what is peculiar to man. Let us exclude, therefore, the life of nutrition and growth. Next there would be a life of perception, but *it* also seems to be shared even by the horse, the ox, and every animal. There remains, then, an active life of the element that has a rational principle; of this, one part has such a principle in the sense of being obedient to one, the other in the sense of possessing one and exercising thought. And, as 'life of the rational element' also has two meanings, we must state that life in the sense of activity is what we mean; for this seems to be the more proper sense of the term. Now if the function of man is an activity of soul which follows or implies a rational principle, and if we say 'a so-and-so' and 'a good so-and-so' have a function which is the same in kind, e.g. a lyre-player and a good lyre-player, and so without qualification in all cases, eminence in respect of goodness being added to the name of the function (for the function of a lyre-player is to play the lyre, and that of a good lyre-player is to do so well): if this is the case [and we state the function of man to be a certain kind of life, and this to be an activity or actions of the soul implying a rational principle, and the function of a good man to be the good and noble performance of these, and if any action is well performed when it is performed in accordance with the appropriate excellence: if this is the case], human good turns out to be activity of soul exhibiting excellence, and if there are more than one excellence, in accordance with the best and most complete.

But we must add 'in a complete life'. For one swallow does not make a summer, nor does one day; and so too one day, or a short time, does not make a man blessed and happy.

Let this serve as an outline of the good; for we must presumably first sketch it roughly, and then later fill in the details. But it would seem that any one is capable of carrying on and articulating what has once been well outlined, and that time is a good discoverer or partner in such a work; to which facts the advances of the arts are due; for any one can add what is lacking. And we must also remember what has been said before,[3] and not look for precision in all things alike, but in each class of things such precision as accords with the subject-matter, and so much as is appropriate to the inquiry. For a carpenter and a geometer investigate the right angle in different ways; the former does so in so far as the right angle is useful for his work, while the latter inquires what it is or what sort of thing it is; for he is a spectator of the truth. We must act in the same way, then, in all other matters as well, that our main task may not be subordinated to minor questions. Nor must we demand the cause in all matters alike; it is enough in some cases that the *fact* be well established, as in the case of the first principles; the fact is a primary thing and first principle. Now of first principles we see some by induction, some by perception, some by a certain habituation, and others too in other ways. But each set of principles we must try to investigate in the natural way, and we must take pains to determine them correctly, since they have a great influence on what follows. For the beginning is thought to be more than half of the whole, and many of the questions we ask are cleared up by it.

Our definition is confirmed by current beliefs about happiness

8.   But we must consider happiness in the light not only of our conclusion and our premises, but also of what is commonly said about it; for with a true view all the data harmonize, but with a false one the facts soon clash. Now goods have been divided into three classes,[4] and some are described as external, others as relating to soul or to body; we call those that relate to soul most properly and truly goods, and psychical actions and activities we class as relating to soul. Therefore our account must be sound, at least according to this view, which is an old one and agreed on by philosophers. It is correct also in that we identify the end with certain actions and activities; for thus it falls among goods of the soul and not among external goods. Another belief which harmonizes with our account is that the happy man lives well and fares well; for we have practically defined happiness as a sort of living and faring well. The characteristics that are looked for in happiness seem also, all of them, to belong to what we have defined happiness as being. For some identify happiness with virtue, some with practical wisdom, others with a kind of philosophic wisdom, others with these, or one of these, accompanied by pleasure or not without pleasure; while others include also external prosperity. Now some of these views have been held by many men and men of old, others by a few eminent persons; and it is not probable that either of these should be entirely mistaken, but rather that they should be right in at least some one respect, or even in most respects.

With those who identify happiness with virtue or some one virtue our account is in harmony; for to virtue belongs virtuous activity. But it makes, perhaps, no small difference whether we place the chief good in possession or in use, in state of mind or in activity. For the state of mind may exist without producing any good result, as in a man who is asleep or in some other way quite inactive, but the activity cannot; for one who has the activity will of necessity be acting, and acting well. And as in the Olympic Games it is not the most beautiful and the strongest that are crowned but those who compete (for it is some of these that are victorious), so those who act win, and rightly win, the noble and good things in life.

Their life is also in itself pleasant. For pleasure is a state of *soul*, and to each man that which he is said to be a lover of is pleasant; e.g. not only is a horse pleasant to the lover of horses, and a spectacle to the lover of sights, but also in the same way just acts are pleasant to the lover of justice and in general virtuous acts to the lover of virtue. Now for most men their pleasures are in conflict with one another because these are not by nature pleasant, but the lovers of what is noble find pleasant the things that are by nature pleasant; and virtuous actions are such, so that these are pleasant for such men as well as in their own nature. Their life, therefore, has no further need of pleasure as a sort of adventitious charm, but has its pleasure in itself. For, besides what we have said, the man who does not rejoice in noble actions is not even good; since no one would call a man just who did not enjoy acting justly, nor any man liberal who did not enjoy liberal actions; and similarly in all other cases. If this is so, virtuous actions must be in themselves pleasant. But they are also *good* and *noble*, and have each of these attributes in the highest degree, since the good man judges well about these attributes; his judgement is such as we have described.[5] Happiness then is the best, noblest, and most pleasant thing in the world, and these attributes are not severed as in the inscription at Delos –

> Most noble is that which is justest, and best is health;
> But most pleasant it is to win what we love.

For all these properties belong to the best activities; and these, or one – the best – of these, we identify with happiness.

Yet evidently, as we said,[6] it needs the external goods as well; for it is impossible, or not easy, to do noble acts without the proper equipment. In many actions we use friends and riches and political power as instruments; and there are some things the lack of which takes the lustre from happiness – good birth, goodly children, beauty; for the man who is very ugly in appearance or ill-born or solitary and childless is not very likely to be happy, and perhaps a man would be still less likely if he had thoroughly bad children or friends or had lost good children or friends by death. As we said,[7] then, happiness seems to need this sort of prosperity in addition; for which reason some identify happiness with good fortune, though others identify it with virtue.

Notes

1 Strictly, double-reed instruments.
2 i. 10, 11, ix. 10.

3   1094^b11–27.
4   Pl. *Euthyd.* 279 AB, *Phil.* 48 E, *Laws*, 743 E.
5   I.e., he judges that virtuous actions are good and noble in the highest degree.
6   1098^b26–29.
7   Ibid.

Book II – Moral Virtue

Moral virtue, how produced, in what medium and in what manner exhibited

Moral virtue, like the arts, is acquired by repetition of the corresponding acts

1. Virtue, then, being of two kinds, intellectual and moral, intellectual virtue in the main owes both its birth and its growth to teaching (for which reason it requires experience and time), while moral virtue comes about as a result of habit, whence also its name (ἠθική) is one that is formed by a slight variation from the word ἔθος (habit). From this it is also plain that none of the moral virtues arises in us by nature; for nothing that exists by nature can form a habit contrary to its nature. For instance the stone which by nature moves downwards cannot be habituated to move upwards, not even if one tries to train it by throwing it up ten thousand times; nor can fire be habituated to move downwards, nor can anything else that by nature behaves in one way be trained to behave in another. Neither by nature, then, nor contrary to nature do the virtues arise in us; rather we are adapted by nature to receive them, and are made perfect by habit.

Again, of all the things that come to us by nature we first acquire the potentiality and later exhibit the activity (this is plain in the case of the senses; for it was not by often seeing or often hearing that we got these senses, but on the contrary we had them before we used them, and did not come to have them by using them); but the virtues we get by first exercising them, as also happens in the case of the arts as well. For the things we have to learn before we can do them, we learn by doing them, e.g. men become builders by building and lyre-players by playing the lyre; so too we become just by doing just acts, temperate by doing temperate acts, brave by doing brave acts.

This is confirmed by what happens in states; for legislators make the citizens good by forming habits in them, and this is the wish of every legislator, and those who do not effect it miss their mark, and it is in this that a good constitution differs from a bad one.

Again, it is from the same causes and by the same means that every virtue is both produced and destroyed, and similarly every art; for it is from playing the lyre that both good and bad lyre-players are produced. And the corresponding statement is true of builders and of all the rest; men will be good or bad builders as a result of building well or badly. For if this were not so, there would have been no need of a teacher, but all men would have been born good or bad at their craft. This, then, is the case with the virtues also; by doing the acts that we do in our transactions with other men we become just or unjust, and by doing the acts that we do in the presence of danger, and by being habituated to feel fear or confidence, we become brave or cowardly. The same is true of appetites and feelings of anger; some men become temperate and good-tempered, others self-indulgent and irascible, by behaving in one way or the other in the appropriate circumstances. Thus, in one word, states of character arise out of like activities. This is why the activities we exhibit must be of a certain kind; it is because the states of character correspond to the differences between these. It makes no small difference, then, whether we form habits of one kind or of another from our very youth; it makes a very great difference, or rather *all* the difference.

These acts cannot be prescribed exactly, but must avoid excess and defect

2.   Since, then, the present inquiry does not aim at theoretical knowledge like the others (for we are inquiring not in order to know what virtue is, but in order to become good, since otherwise our inquiry would have been of no use), we must examine the nature of actions, namely how we ought to do them; for these determine also the nature of the states of character that are produced, as we have said.[1] Now, that we must act according to the right rule is a common principle and must be assumed – it will be discussed later,[2] i.e. both what the right rule is, and how it is related to the other virtues. But this must be agreed upon beforehand, that the whole account of matters of conduct must be given in outline and not precisely, as we said at the very beginning[3] that the accounts we demand must be in accordance with the subject-matter; matters concerned with conduct and questions of what is good for us have no fixity, any more than matters of health. The general account being of this nature, the account of particular cases is yet more lacking in exactness; for they do not fall under any art or precept, but the agents themselves must in each case consider what is appropriate to the occasion, as happens also in the art of medicine or of navigation.

But though our present account is of this nature we must give what help we can. First, then, let us consider this, that it is the nature of such things to be destroyed by defect and excess, as we see in the case of strength and of health (for to gain light on things imperceptible we must use the evidence of sensible things); exercise either excessive or defective destroys the strength, and similarly drink or food which is above or below a certain amount destroys the health, while that which is proportionate both produces and increases and preserves it. So too is it, then, in the case of temperance and courage and the other virtues. For the man who flies from and fears everything and does not stand his ground against anything becomes a coward, and the man who fears nothing at all but goes to meet every danger becomes rash; and similarly the man who indulges in every pleasure and abstains from none becomes self-indulgent, while the man who shuns every pleasure, as boors do, becomes in a way insensible; temperance and courage, then, are destroyed by excess and defect, and preserved by the mean.

But not only are the sources and causes of their origination and growth the same as those of their destruction, but also the sphere of their actualization will be the same; for this is also true of the things which are more evident to sense, e.g. of strength; it is produced by taking much food and undergoing much exertion, and it is the strong man that will be most able to do these things. So too is it with the virtues; by abstaining from pleasures we become temperate, and it is when we have become so that we are most able to abstain from them; and similarly too in the case of courage; for by being habituated to despise things that are fearful and to stand our ground against them we become brave, and it is when we have become so that we shall be most able to stand our ground against them.

Pleasure in doing virtuous acts is a sign that the virtuous disposition has been acquired: a variety of considerations show the essential connexion of moral virtue with pleasure and pain

3.   We must take as a sign of states of character the pleasure or pain that supervenes upon acts; for the man who abstains from bodily pleasures and delights in this very fact is temperate, while the man who is annoyed at it is self-indulgent, and he who stands his ground against things that are terrible and delights in this or at least is not pained is brave, while the man who is pained is a coward. For moral excellence is concerned with pleasures and pains; it is on account of the pleasure that we do bad things, and on account of the pain that we abstain from noble ones. Hence we ought to have been brought up in a particular way from our very youth, as Plato says,[4] so as both to delight in and to be pained by the things that we ought; this is the right education.

Again, if the virtues are concerned with actions and passions, and every passion and every action is accompanied by pleasure and pain, for this reason also virtue will be concerned with pleasures and pains. This is indicated also by the fact that punishment is inflicted by these means; for it is a kind of cure, and it is the nature of cures to be effected by contraries.

Again, as we said but lately,[5] every state of soul has a nature relative to and concerned with the kind of things by which it tends to be made worse or better; but it is by reason of pleasures and pains that men become bad, by pursuing and avoiding these – either the pleasures and pains they ought not or when they ought not or as they ought not, or by going wrong in one of the other similar ways that may be distinguished. Hence men[6] even define the virtues as certain states of impassivity and rest; not well, however, because they speak absolutely, and do not say 'as one ought' and 'as one ought not' and 'when one ought or ought not', and the other things that may be added. We assume, then, that this kind of excellence tends to do what is best with regard to pleasures and pains, and vice does the contrary.

The following facts also may show us that virtue and vice are concerned with these same things. There being three objects of choice and three of avoidance, the noble, the advantageous, the pleasant, and their contraries, the base, the injurious, the painful, about all of these the good man tends to go right and the bad man to go wrong, and especially about pleasure; for this is common to the animals, and also it accompanies all objects of choice; for even the noble and the advantageous appear pleasant.

Again, it has grown up with us all from our infancy; this is why it is difficult to rub off this passion, engrained as it is in our life. And we measure even our actions, some of us more and others less, by the rule of pleasure and pain. For this reason, then, our whole inquiry must be about these; for to feel delight and pain rightly or wrongly has no small effect on our actions.

Again, it is harder to fight with pleasure than with anger, to use Heraclitus' phrase, but both art and virtue are always concerned with what is harder; for even the good is better when it is harder. Therefore for this reason also the whole concern both of virtue and of political science is with pleasures and pains; for the man who uses these well will be good, he who uses them badly bad.

That virtue, then, is concerned with pleasures and pains, and that by the acts from which it arises it is both increased and, if they are done differently, destroyed, and that the acts from which it arose are those in which it actualizes itself – let this be taken as said.

The actions that produce moral virtue are not good in the same sense as those that flow from it: the latter must fulfil certain conditions not necessary in the case of the arts

4.   The question might be asked, what we mean by saying[7] that we must become just by doing just acts, and temperate by doing temperate acts; for if men do just and temperate acts, they are already just and temperate, exactly as, if they do what is in accordance with the laws of grammar and of music, they are grammarians and musicians.

Or is this not true even of the arts? It is possible to do something that is in accordance with the laws of grammar, either by chance or under the guidance of another. A man will be a grammarian, then, only when he has both said something grammatical and said it grammatically; and this means doing it in accordance with the grammatical knowledge in himself.

Again, the case of the arts and that of the virtues are not similar; for the products of the arts have their goodness in themselves, so that it is enough that they should have a certain character, but if the acts that are in accordance with the virtues have themselves a certain character it does not follow that they are done justly or temperately. The agent also must be in a certain condition when he does them; in the first place he must have knowledge, secondly he must choose the acts, and choose them for their own sakes, and thirdly his action must proceed from a firm and unchangeable character. These are not reckoned in as conditions of the possession of the arts, except the bare knowledge; but as a condition of the possession of the virtues knowledge has little or no weight, while the other conditions count not for a little but for everything, i.e. the very conditions which result from often doing just and temperate acts.

Actions, then, are called just and temperate when they are such as the just or the temperate man would do; but it is not the man who does these that is just and temperate, but the man who also does them *as* just and temperate men do them. It is well said, then, that it is by doing just acts that the just man is produced, and by doing temperate acts the temperate man; without doing these no one would have even a prospect of becoming good.

But most people do not do these, but take refuge in theory and think they are being philosophers and will become good in this way, behaving somewhat like patients who listen attentively to their doctors, but do none of the things they are ordered to do. As the latter will not be made well in body by such a course of treatment, the former will not be made well in soul by such a course of philosophy.

Definition of moral virtue

The genus of moral virtue: it is a state of character, not a passion, nor a faculty

5.   Next we must consider what virtue is. Since things that are found in the soul are of three kinds – passions, faculties, states of character – virtue must be one of these. By passions I mean appetite, anger, fear, confidence, envy, joy, friendly feeling, hatred, longing, emulation, pity, and in general the feelings that are accompanied by pleasure or pain; by faculties the things in virtue of which we are said to be capable of feeling these, e.g. of becoming angry or being pained or feeling pity; by states of character the things in virtue of which we stand well or badly with reference to the passions, e.g. with reference to anger we stand badly if we feel it violently or too weakly, and well if we feel it moderately; and similarly with reference to the other passions.

Now neither the virtues nor the vices are *passions*, because we are not called good or bad on the ground of our passions, but are so called on the ground of our virtues and our vices, and because we are neither praised nor blamed for our passions (for the man who feels fear or anger is not praised, nor is the man who simply feels anger blamed, but the man who feels it in a certain way), but for our virtues and our vices we *are* praised or blamed.

Again, we feel anger and fear without choice, but the virtues are modes of choice or involve choice. Further, in respect of the passions we are said to be moved, but in respect of the virtues and the vices we are said not to be moved but to be disposed in a particular way.

For these reasons also they are not *faculties*; for we are neither called good or bad, nor praised or blamed, for the simple capacity of feeling the passions; again, we have the faculties by nature, but we are not made good or bad by nature; we have spoken of this before.[8]

If, then, the virtues are neither passions nor faculties, all that remains is that they should be *states of character*.

Thus we have stated what virtue is in respect of its genus.

The differentia of moral virtue: it is a disposition to choose the mean

6.   We must, however, not only describe virtue as a state of character, but also say what sort of state it is. We may remark, then, that every virtue or excellence both brings into good condition the thing of which it is the excellence and makes the work of that thing be done well; e.g. the excellence of the eye makes both the eye and its work good; for it is by

the excellence of the eye that we see well. Similarly the excellence of the horse makes a horse both good in itself and good at running and at carrying its rider and at awaiting the attack of the enemy. Therefore, if this is true in every case, the virtue of man also will be the state of character which makes a man good and which makes him do his own work well.

How this is to happen we have stated already,[9] but it will be made plain also by the following consideration of the specific nature of virtue. In everything that is continuous and divisible it is possible to take more, less, or an equal amount, and that either in terms of the thing itself or relatively to us; and the equal is an intermediate between excess and defect. By the intermediate in the object I mean that which is equidistant from each of the extremes, which is one and the same for all men; by the intermediate relatively to us that which is neither too much nor too little – and this is not one, nor the same for all. For instance, if ten is many and two is few, six is the intermediate, taken in terms of the object; for it exceeds and is exceeded by an equal amount; this is intermediate according to arithmetical proportion. But the intermediate relatively to us is not to be taken so; if ten pounds are too much for a particular person to eat and two too little, it does not follow that the trainer will order six pounds; for this also is perhaps too much for the person who is to take it, or too little – too little for Milo,[10] too much for the beginner in athletic exercises. The same is true of running and wrestling. Thus a master of any art avoids excess and defect, but seeks the intermediate and chooses this – the intermediate not in the object but relatively to us.

If it is thus, then, that every art does its work well – by looking to the intermediate and judging its works by this standard (so that we often say of good works of art that it is not possible either to take away or to add anything, implying that excess and defect destroy the goodness of works of art, while the mean preserves it; and good artists, as we say, look to this in their work), and if, further, virtue is more exact and better than any art, as nature also is, then virtue must have the quality of aiming at the intermediate. I mean moral virtue; for it is this that is concerned with passions and actions, and in these there is excess, defect, and the intermediate. For instance, both fear and confidence and appetite and anger and pity and in general pleasure and pain may be felt both too much and too little, and in both cases not well; but to feel them at the right times, with reference to the right objects, towards the right people, with the right motive, and in the right way, is what is both intermediate and best, and this is characteristic of virtue. Similarly with regard to actions also there is excess, defect, and the intermediate. Now virtue is concerned with passions and actions, in which excess is a form of failure, and so is defect, while the intermediate is praised and is a form of success; and being praised and being successful are both characteristics of virtue. Therefore virtue is a kind of mean, since, as we have seen, it aims at what is intermediate.

Again, it is possible to fail in many ways (for evil belongs to the class of the unlimited, as the Pythagoreans conjectured, and good to that of the limited), while to succeed is possible only in one way (for which reason also one is easy and the other difficult – to miss the mark easy, to hit it difficult); for these reasons also, then, excess and defect are characteristic of vice, and the mean of virtue;

For men are good in but one way, but bad in many.

Virtue, then, is a state of character concerned with choice, lying in a mean, i.e. the mean relative to us, this being determined by a rational principle, and by that principle by which the man of practical wisdom would determine it. Now it is a mean between two vices, that which depends on excess and that which depends on defect; and again it is a mean because the vices respectively fall short of or exceed what is right in both passions and actions, while virtue both finds and chooses that which is intermediate. Hence in respect of what it is, i.e. the definition which states its essence, virtue is a mean, with regard to what is best and right an extreme.

But not every action nor every passion admits of a mean; for some have names that already imply badness, e.g. spite, shamelessness, envy, and in the case of actions adultery, theft, murder; for all of these and suchlike things imply by their names that they are themselves bad, and not the excesses or deficiencies of them. It is not possible, then, ever to be right with regard to them; one must always be wrong. Nor does goodness or badness with regard to such things depend on committing adultery with the right woman, at the right time, and in the right way, but simply to do any of them is to go wrong. It would be equally absurd, then, to expect that in unjust, cowardly, and voluptuous action there should be a mean, an excess, and a deficiency; for at that rate there would be a mean of excess and of deficiency, an excess of excess, and a deficiency of deficiency. But as there is no excess and deficiency of temperance and courage because what is intermediate is in a sense an extreme, so too of the actions we have mentioned there is no mean nor any excess and deficiency, but however they are done they are wrong; for in general there is neither a mean of excess and deficiency, nor excess and deficiency of a mean.

The above proposition illustrated by reference to particular virtues

7.   We must, however, not only make this general statement, but also apply it to the individual facts. For among statements about conduct those which are general apply more widely, but those which are particular are more true, since conduct has to do with individual cases, and our statements must harmonize with the facts in these cases. We may take these cases from our table. With regard to feelings of fear and confidence courage is the mean; of the people who exceed, he who exceeds in fearlessness has no name (many of the states have no name), while the man who exceeds in confidence is rash, and he who exceeds in fear and falls short in confidence is a coward. With regard to pleasures and pains – not all of them, and not so much with regard to the pains – the mean is temperance, the excess self-indulgence. Persons deficient with regard to the pleasures are not often found; hence such persons also have received no name. But let us call them 'insensible'.

With regard to giving and taking of money the mean is liberality, the excess and the defect prodigality and meanness. In these actions people exceed and fall short in contrary ways; the prodigal exceeds in spending and falls short in taking, while the mean man exceeds in taking and falls short in spending. (At present we are giving a mere outline or summary, and are satisfied with this; later these states will be more exactly determined.)[11] With regard to money there are also other dispositions – a mean, magnificence (for the magnificent man differs from the liberal man; the former deals with large sums, the latter with small ones), an excess, tastelessness and vulgarity, and a deficiency, niggardliness; these differ from the states opposed to liberality, and the mode of their difference will be stated later.[12]

With regard to honour and dishonour the mean is proper pride, the excess is known as a sort of 'empty vanity', and the deficiency is undue humility; and as we said[13] liberality was related to magnificence, differing from it by dealing with small sums, so there is a state similarly related to proper pride, being concerned with small honours while that is concerned with great. For it is possible to desire honour as one ought, and more than one ought, and less, and the man who exceeds in his desires is called ambitious, the man who falls short unambitious, while the intermediate person has no name. The dispositions also are nameless, except that that of the ambitious man is called ambition. Hence the people who are at the extremes lay claim to the middle place; and we ourselves sometimes call the intermediate person ambitious and sometimes unambitious, and sometimes praise the ambitious man and sometimes the unambitious. The reason of our doing this will be stated in what follows;[14] but now let us speak of the remaining states according to the method which has been indicated.

With regard to anger also there is an excess, a deficiency, and a mean. Although they can scarcely be said to have names, yet since we call the intermediate person good-tempered let us call the mean good temper; of the persons at the extremes let the one who exceeds be called irascible, and his vice irascibility, and the man who falls short an unirascible sort of person, and the deficiency unirascibility.

There are also three other means, which have a certain likeness to one another, but differ from one another: for they are all concerned with intercourse in words and actions, but differ in that one is concerned with truth in this sphere, the other two with pleasantness; and of this one kind is exhibited in giving amusement, the other in all the circumstances of life. We must therefore speak of these too, that we may the better see that in all things the mean is praiseworthy, and the extremes neither praise-worthy nor right, but worthy of blame. Now most of these states also have no names, but we must try, as in the other cases, to invent names ourselves so that we may be clear and easy to follow. With regard to truth, then, the intermediate is a truthful sort of person and the mean may be called truthfulness, while the pretence which exaggerates is boastfulness and the person characterized by it a boaster, and that which understates is mock modesty and the person characterized by it mock-modest. With regard to pleasantness in the giving of amusement the intermediate person is ready-witted and the disposition ready wit, the excess is buffoonery and the person characterized by it a buffoon, while the man who falls short is a sort of boor and his state is boorishness. With regard to the remaining kind of pleasantness, that which is exhibited in life in general, the man who is pleasant in the right way is friendly and the mean is friendliness, while the man who exceeds is an obsequious person if he has no end in view, a flatterer if he is aiming at his own advantage, and the man who falls short and is unpleasant in all circumstances is a quarrelsome and surly sort of person.

There are also means in the passions and concerned with the passions; since shame is not a virtue, and yet praise is extended to the modest man. For even in these matters one man is said to be intermediate, and another to exceed, as for instance the bashful man who is ashamed of everything; while he who falls short or is not ashamed of anything at all is shameless, and the intermediate person is modest. Righteous indignation is a mean between envy and spite, and these states are concerned with the pain and pleasure that are felt at the fortunes of our neighbours; the man who is characterized by righteous indignation is pained at undeserved good fortune, the envious man, going beyond him, is pained at all good fortune, and the spiteful man falls so far short of being pained that he even rejoices.[15] But these states there will be an opportunity of describing elsewhere;[16] with regard to justice, since it has not one simple meaning, we shall, after describing the other states, distinguish its two kinds and say how each of them is a mean;[17] and similarly we shall treat also of the rational virtues.[18]

Characteristics of the extreme and mean states: practical corollaries

The extremes are opposed to each other and to the mean

8.   There are three kinds of disposition, then, two of them vices, involving excess and deficiency respectively, and one a virtue, viz. the mean, and all are in a sense opposed to all; for the extreme states are contrary both to the intermediate state and to each other, and the intermediate to the extremes; as the equal is greater relatively to the less, less relatively to the greater, so the middle states are excessive relatively to the deficiencies, deficient relatively to the excesses, both in passions and in actions. For the brave man appears rash relatively to the coward, and cowardly relatively to the rash man; and similarly the temperate man appears self-indulgent relatively to the insensible man, insensible relatively to the self-indulgent, and the liberal man prodigal relatively to the mean man, mean relatively to the prodigal. Hence also the people at the extremes push the intermediate man each over to the other, and the brave man is called rash by the coward, cowardly by the rash man, and correspondingly in the other cases.

These states being thus opposed to one another, the greatest contrariety is that of the extremes to each other, rather than to the intermediate; for these are further from each other than from the intermediate, as the great is further from the small and the small from the great than both are from the equal. Again, to the intermediate some extremes show a certain likeness, as that of rashness to courage and that of prodigality to liberality; but the extremes show the greatest unlikeness to each other; now contraries are defined as the things that are furthest from each other, so that things that are further apart are more contrary.

To the mean in some cases the deficiency, in some the excess, is more opposed; e.g. it is not rashness, which is an excess, but cowardice, which is a deficiency, that is more opposed to courage, and not insensibility, which is a deficiency, but self-indulgence, which is an excess, that is more opposed to temperance. This happens from two reasons, one being drawn from the thing itself; for because one extreme is nearer and liker to the intermediate, we oppose not this but rather its contrary to the intermediate. E.g., since rashness is thought liker and nearer to courage, and cowardice more unlike, we oppose rather the latter to courage; for things that are further from the intermediate are thought more contrary to it. This, then, is one cause, drawn from the thing itself; another is drawn from ourselves; for the things to which we ourselves more naturally tend seem more contrary to the intermediate. For instance, we ourselves tend more naturally to pleasures, and hence are more easily carried away towards self-indulgence than towards propriety. We describe as contrary to the mean, then, rather the directions in which we more often go to great lengths; and therefore self-indulgence, which is an excess, is the more contrary to temperance.

The mean is hard to attain, and is grasped by perception, not by reasoning

9.   That moral virtue is a mean, then, and in what sense it is so, and that it is a mean between two vices, the one involving excess, the other deficiency, and that it is such because its character is to aim at what is intermediate in passions and in actions, has been sufficiently stated. Hence also it is no easy task to be good. For in everything it is no easy task to find the middle, e.g. to find the middle of a circle is not for everyone but for him who knows; so, too, anyone can get angry – that is easy – or give or spend money; but to do this to the right person, to the right extent, at the right time, with the right motive, and in the right way, *that* is not for everyone, nor is it easy; wherefore goodness is both rare and laudable and noble.

Hence he who aims at the intermediate must first depart from what is the more contrary to it, as Calypso advises –

Hold the ship out beyond that surf and spray.[19]

For of the extremes one is more erroneous, one less so; therefore, since to hit the mean is hard in the extreme, we must as a second best, as people say, take the least of the evils; and this will be done best in the way we describe.

But we must consider the things towards which we ourselves also are easily carried away; for some of us tend to one thing, some to another; and this will be recognizable from the pleasure and the pain we feel. We must drag ourselves away to the contrary extreme; for we shall get into the intermediate state by drawing well away from error, as people do in straightening sticks that are bent.

Now in everything the pleasant or pleasure is most to be guarded against; for we do not judge it impartially. We ought, then, to feel towards pleasure as the elders of the people felt towards Helen, and in all circumstances repeat their saying;[20] for if we dismiss pleasure thus we are less likely to go astray. It is by doing this, then, (to sum the matter up) that we shall best be able to hit the mean.

But this is no doubt difficult, and especially in individual cases; for it is not easy to determine both how and with whom and on what provocation and how long one should be angry; for we too sometimes praise those who fall short and call them good-tempered, but sometimes we praise those who get angry and call them manly. The man, however, who deviates little from goodness is not blamed, whether he do so in the direction of the more or of the less, but only the man who deviates more widely; for *he* does not fail to be noticed. But up to what point and to what extent a man must deviate before he becomes blameworthy it is not easy to determine by reasoning, any more than anything else that is perceived by the senses; such things depend on particular facts, and the decision rests with perception. So much, then, is plain, that the intermediate state is in all things to be praised, but that we must incline sometimes towards the excess, sometimes towards the deficiency; for so shall we most easily hit the mean and what is right.

Notes

1   [a]31–[b]25.
2   vi. 13.
3   1094[b]11–27.
4   *Laws*, 653 A ff., *Rep.* 401 E–402 A.
5   [a]27–[b]3.
6   Probably Speusippus is referred to.
7   1103[a]31–[b]25, 1104[a]27–[b]3.
8   1103[a]18–[b]2.
9   1104[a]11–27.
10   A famous athlete.
11   v. 1.
12   1122[a]20–29, [b]10–18.
13   ll. 17–19.
14   [b]11–26, 1125[b]14–18.
15   Aristotle must mean that while the envious man is pained at the good fortune

of others, whether deserved or not, the spiteful man is pleased at the *bad* fortune of others, whether deserved or not. But if he had stated this in full, he would have seen that there is no real opposition.

16 The reference may be to the whole treatment of the moral virtues in iii. 6–iv. 9, or to the discussion of shame in iv. 9 and an intended corresponding discussion of righteous indignation, or to the discussion of these two states in *Rhet.* ii. 6, 9, 10.

17 1129^a26-^b1, 1130^a14-^b5, 1131^b9-15, 1132^a24-30, $1133^b30-1134^a1$.

18 Bk. vi.

19 *Od.* xii. 219 f. (Mackail's trans.). But it was Circe who gave the advice (xii. 108), and the actual quotation is from Odysseus' orders to his steersman.

20 *Il.* iii. 156–60.

Book III, 6–12

Courage

Courage concerned with the feelings of fear and confidence – strictly speaking, with the fear of death in battle

6. That it is a mean with regard to feelings of fear and confidence has already been made evident;[1] and plainly the things we fear are fearful things, and these are, to speak without qualification, evils; for which reason people even define fear as expectation of evil. Now we fear all evils, e.g. disgrace, poverty, disease, friendlessness, death, but the brave man is not thought to be concerned with all; for to fear some things is even right and noble, and it is base not to fear them – e.g. disgrace; he who fears this is good and modest, and he who does not is shameless. He is, however, by some people called brave, by a transference of the word to a new meaning; for he has in him something which is like the brave man, since the brave man also is a fearless person. Poverty and disease we perhaps ought not to fear, nor in general the things that do not proceed from vice and are not due to a man himself. But not even the man who is fearless of these is brave. Yet we apply the word to him also in virtue of a similarity; for some who in the dangers of war are cowards are liberal and are confident in face of the loss of money. Nor is a man a coward if he fears insult to his wife and children or envy or anything of the kind; nor brave if he is confident when he is about to be flogged. With what sort of fearful things, then, is the brave man concerned? Surely with the greatest; for no one is more likely than he to stand his ground against what is awe-inspiring. Now death is the most fearful of all things; for it is the end, and nothing is thought to be any longer either good or bad for the dead. But the brave man would not seem to be concerned even with death in *all* circumstances, e.g. at sea or in disease. In what circumstances, then? Surely in the noblest. Now such deaths are those in battle; for these take place in the greatest and noblest danger. And these are correspondingly honoured in city-states and at the courts of monarchs. Properly, then, he will be called brave who is fearless in face of a noble death, and of all emergencies that involve death; and the emergencies of war are in the highest degree of this kind. Yet at sea also, and in disease, the brave man is fearless, but not in the same way as the seamen; for he has given up hope of safety, and is disliking the thought of death in this shape, while they are hopeful because of their experience. At the same time, we show courage in situations where there is the opportunity of showing prowess or where death is noble; but in these forms of death neither of these conditions is fulfilled.

The motive of courage is the sense of honour: characteristics of the opposite vices, cowardice and rashness

7. What is fearful is not the same for all men; but we say there are things fearful even beyond human strength. These, then, are fearful to every one – at least to every sensible man; but the fearful things that are *not* beyond human strength differ in magnitude and degree, and so too do the things that inspire confidence. Now the brave man is as dauntless as man may be. Therefore, while he will fear even the things that are not beyond human strength, he will face them as he ought and as the rule directs, for honour's sake; for this is the end of virtue. But it is possible to fear these more, or less, and again to fear things that are not fearful as if they were. Of the faults that are committed, one consists in fearing what we should not, another in fearing as we should not, another in fearing when we should not, and so on; and so too with respect to the things that inspire confidence. The man, then, who faces and who fears the right things and from the right motive, in the right way and at the right time, and who feels confidence under the corresponding conditions, is brave; for the brave man feels and acts according to the merits of the case and in whatever way the rule directs. Now the end of every activity is conformity to the corresponding state of character. This is true, therefore, of the brave man as well as of others. But courage is noble. Therefore the end also is noble; for each thing is defined by its end. Therefore it is for a noble end that the brave man endures and acts as courage directs.

Of those who go to excess he who exceeds in fearlessness has no name (we have said previously that many states of character have no names),[2] but he would be a sort of madman or insensitive to pain if he feared nothing, neither earthquakes nor the waves, as they say the Celts do not; while the man who exceeds in confidence about what really is fearful is rash. The rash man, however, is also thought to be boastful and only a pretender to courage; at all events, as the brave man *is* with regard to what is fearful, so the rash man wishes to *appear*; and so he imitates him in situations where he can. Hence also most of them are a mixture of rashness and cowardice; for, while in these situations they display confidence, they do not hold their ground against what is really fearful. The man who exceeds in fear is a coward; for he fears both what he ought not and as he ought not, and all the similar characterizations attach to him. He is lacking also in confidence; but he is more conspicuous for his excess of fear in painful situations. The coward, then, is a despairing sort of person; for he fears everything. The brave man, on the other hand, has the opposite disposition; for confidence is the mark of a hopeful disposition. The coward, the rash man, and the brave man, then, are concerned with the same objects but are differently disposed towards them; for the first two exceed and fall short, while the third holds the middle, which is the right, position; and rash men are precipitate, and wish for dangers beforehand but draw back when they are in them, while brave men are excited in the moment of action, but collected beforehand.

As we have said, then, courage is a mean with respect to things that inspire confidence or fear, in the circumstances that have been stated;[3] and it chooses or endures things because it is noble to do so, or because it is base not to do so.[4] But to die to escape from poverty or love or anything painful is not the mark of a brave man, but rather of a coward; for it is softness to fly from what is troublesome, and such a man endures death not because it is noble but to fly from evil.

Five kinds of courage improperly so called

8.   Courage, then, is something of this sort, but the name is also applied to five other kinds. (1) First comes the courage of the citizen-soldier; for this is most like true courage. Citizen-soldiers seem to face dangers because of the penalties imposed by the laws and the reproaches they would otherwise incur, and because of the honours they win by such action; and therefore those peoples seem to be bravest among whom cowards are held in dishonour and brave men in honour. This is the kind of courage that Homer depicts, e.g. in Diomede and in Hector:

First will Polydamas be to heap reproach on me then;[5]

and

> For Hector one day 'mid the Trojans shall utter
> his vaunting harangue:
> 'Afraid was Tydeides, and fled from my face.'[6]

This kind of courage is most like to that which we described earlier,[7] because it is due to virtue; for it is due to shame and to desire of a noble object (i.e. honour) and avoidance of disgrace, which is ignoble. One might rank in the same class even those who are compelled by their rulers; but they are inferior, inasmuch as they do what they do not from shame but from fear, and to avoid not what is disgraceful but what is painful; for their masters compel them, as Hector[8] does:

> But if I shall spy any dastard that cowers far from
> the fight,
> Vainly will such an one hope to escape from the dogs.

And those who give them their posts, and beat them if they retreat, do the same, and so do those who draw them up with trenches or something of the sort behind them; all of these apply compulsion. But one ought to be brave not under compulsion but because it is noble to be so.

(2)   Experience with regard to particular facts is also thought to be courage; this is indeed the reason why Socrates thought courage was knowledge. Other people exhibit this quality in other dangers, and professional soldiers exhibit it in the dangers of war; for there seem to be many empty alarms in war, of which these have had the most comprehensive experience; therefore they seem brave, because the others do not know the nature of the facts. Again, their experience makes them most capable in attack and in defence, since they can use their arms and have the kind that are likely to be best both for attack and for defence; therefore they fight like armed men against unarmed or like trained athletes against amateurs; for in such contests too it is not the bravest men that fight best, but those who are strongest and have their bodies in the best condition. Professional soldiers turn cowards, however, when the danger puts too great a strain on them and they are inferior in numbers and equipment; for they are the first to fly, while citizen-forces die at their posts, as in fact happened at the temple of Hermes.[9] For to the latter flight

is disgraceful and death is preferable to safety on those terms; while the former from the very beginning faced the danger on the assumption that they were stronger, and when they know the facts they fly, fearing death more than disgrace; but the brave man is not that sort of person.

(3) Passion also is sometimes reckoned as courage; those who act from passion, like wild beasts rushing at those who have wounded them, are thought to be brave, because brave men also are passionate; for passion above all things is eager to rush on danger, and hence Homer's 'put strength into his passion'[10] and 'aroused their spirit and passion'[11] and 'hard he breathed panting'[12] and 'his blood boiled'.[13] For all such expressions seem to indicate the stirring and onset of passion. Now brave men act for honour's sake, but passion aids them; while wild beasts act under the influence of pain; for they attack because they have been wounded or because they are afraid, since if they are in a forest they do not come near one. Thus they are not brave because, driven by pain and passion, they rush on danger without foreseeing any of the perils, since at that rate even asses would be brave when they are hungry; for blows will not drive them from their food; and lust also makes adulterers do many daring things. Those creatures are not brave, then, which are driven on to danger by pain or passion. The 'courage' that is due to passion seems to be the most natural, and to be courage if choice and motive be added.

Men, then, as well as beasts, suffer pain when they are angry, and are pleased when they exact their revenge; those who fight for these reasons, however, are pugnacious but not brave; for they do not act for honour's sake nor as the rule directs, but from strength of feeling; they have, however, something akin to courage.

(4) Nor are sanguine people brave; for they are confident in danger only because they have conquered often and against many foes. Yet they closely resemble brave men, because both are confident; but brave men are confident for the reasons stated earlier,[14] while these are so because they think they are the strongest and can suffer nothing. (Drunken men also behave in this way; they become sanguine.) When their adventures do not succeed, however, they run away; but it was[15] the mark of a brave man to face things that are, and seem, terrible for a man, because it is noble to do so and disgraceful not to do so. Hence also it is thought the mark of a braver man to be fearless and undisturbed in sudden alarms than to be so in those that are foreseen; for it must have proceeded more from a state of character, because less from preparation; acts that are foreseen may be chosen by calculation and rule, but sudden actions must be in accordance with one's state of character.

(5)   People who are ignorant of the danger also appear brave, and they are not far removed from those of a sanguine temper, but are inferior inasmuch as they have no self-reliance while these have. Hence also the sanguine hold their ground for a time; but those who have been deceived about the facts fly if they know or suspect that these are different from what they supposed, as happened to the Argives when they fell in with the Spartans and took them for Sicyonians.[16]

9.   We have, then, described the character both of brave men and of those who are thought to be brave.

Relation of courage to pain and pleasure

Though courage is concerned with confidence and fear, it is not concerned with both alike, but more with the things that inspire fear; for he who is undisturbed in face of these and bears himself as he should towards these is more truly brave than the man who does so towards the things that inspire confidence. It is for facing what is painful, then, as has been said,[17] that men are called brave. Hence also courage involves pain, and is justly praised; for it is harder to face what is painful than to abstain from what is pleasant. Yet the end which courage sets before itself would seem to be pleasant, but to be concealed by the attending circumstances, as happens also in athletic contests; for the end at which boxers aim is pleasant – the crown and the honours – but the blows they take are distressing to flesh and blood, and painful, and so is their whole exertion; and because the blows and the exertions are many the end, which is but small, appears to have nothing pleasant in it. And so, if the case of courage is similar, death and wounds will be painful to the brave man and against his will, but he will face them because it is noble to do so or because it is base not to do so. And the more he is possessed of virtue in its entirety and the happier he is, the more he will be pained at the thought of death; for life is best worth living for such a man, and he is knowingly losing the greatest goods, and this is painful. But he is none the less brave, and perhaps all the more so, because he chooses noble deeds of war at that cost. It is not the case, then, with all the virtues that the exercise of them is pleasant, except in so far as it attains its end. But it is quite possible that the best soldiers may be not men of this sort but those who are less brave but have no other good; for these are ready to face danger, and they sell their life for trifling gains.

So much, then, for courage; it is not difficult to grasp its nature in outline, at any rate, from what has been said.

Temperance

Temperance is limited to certain pleasures of touch

10. After courage let us speak of temperance; for these seem to be the virtues of the irrational parts. We have said[18] that temperance is a mean with regard to pleasures (for it is less, and not in the same way, concerned with pains); self-indulgence also is manifested in the same sphere. Now, therefore, let us determine with what sort of pleasures they are concerned. We may assume the distinction between bodily pleasures and those of the soul, such as love of honour and love of learning; for the lover of each of these delights in that of which he is a lover, the body being in no way affected, but rather the mind; but men who are concerned with such pleasures are called neither temperate nor self-indulgent. Nor, again, are those who are concerned with the other pleasures that are not bodily; for those who are fond of hearing and telling stories and who spend their days on anything that turns up are gossips, but not self-indulgent, nor are those who are pained at the loss of money or of friends.

Temperance must be concerned with bodily pleasures, but not all even of these; for those who delight in objects of vision, such as colours and shapes and painting, are called neither temperate nor self-indulgent; yet it would seem possible to delight even in these either as one should or to excess or to a deficient degree.

And so too is it with objects of hearing; no one calls those who delight extravagantly in music or acting self-indulgent, nor those who do so as they ought temperate.

Nor do we apply these names to those who delight in odour, unless it be incidentally; we do not call those self-indulgent who delight in the odour of apples or roses or incense, but rather those who delight in the odour of unguents or of dainty dishes; for self-indulgent people delight in these because these remind them of the objects of their appetite. And one may see even other people, when they are hungry, delighting in the smell of food; but to delight in this kind of thing is the mark of the self-indulgent man; for these are objects of appetite to him.

Nor is there in animals other than man any pleasure connected with these senses, except incidentally. For dogs do not delight in the scent of hares, but in the eating of them, but the scent told them the hares were there; nor does the lion delight in the lowing of the ox, but in eating it; but he perceived by the lowing that it was near, and therefore appears to delight in the lowing; and similarly he does not delight because he sees 'a stag or a wild goat',[19] but because he is going to make a meal of it.

Temperance and self-indulgence, however, are concerned with the kind of pleasures that the other animals share in, which therefore appear slavish and brutish; these are touch and taste. But even of taste they appear to make little or no use; for the business of taste is the discriminating of flavours, which is done by wine-tasters and people who season dishes; but they hardly take pleasure in making these discriminations, or at least self-indulgent people do not, but in the actual enjoyment, which in all cases comes through touch, both in the case of food and in that of drink and in that of sexual intercourse. This is why a certain gourmand prayed that his throat might become longer than a crane's, implying that it was the contact that he took pleasure in. Thus the sense with which self-indulgence is connected is the most widely shared of the senses; and self-indulgence would seem to be justly a matter of reproach, because it attaches to us not as men but as animals. To delight in such things, then, and to love them above all others, is brutish. For even of the pleasures of touch the most refined have been eliminated, e.g. those produced in the gymnasium by rubbing and by the consequent heat; for the contact characteristic of the self-indulgent man does not affect the whole body but only certain parts.

Characteristics of temperance and its opposites, self-indulgence and 'insensibility'

11.   Of the appetites some seem to be common, others to be peculiar to individuals and acquired; e.g. the appetite for food is natural, since everyone who is without it craves for food or drink, and sometimes for both, and for love also (as Homer says)[20] if he is young and lusty; but not everyone craves for this or that kind of nourishment or love, nor for the same things. Hence such craving appears to be our very own. Yet it has of course something natural about it; for different things are pleasant to different kinds of people, and some things are more pleasant to everyone than chance objects. Now in the natural appetites few go wrong, and only in one direction, that of excess; for to eat or drink whatever offers itself till one is surfeited is to exceed the natural amount, since natural appetite is the replenishment of one's deficiency. Hence these people are called belly-gods, this implying that they fill their belly beyond what is right. It is people of entirely slavish character that become like this. But with regard to the pleasures peculiar to individuals many people go wrong and in many ways. For while the people who are 'fond of so-and-so' are so-called because they delight either in the wrong things, or more than most people do, or in the wrong way, the self-indulgent exceed in all three ways; they both delight in some things that they ought not to delight in (since they are hateful), and if one ought to delight in some of the things they delight in, they do so more than one ought and than most men do.

Plainly, then, excess with regard to pleasures is self-indulgence and is culpable; with regard to pains one is not, as in the case of courage, called temperate for facing them or self-indulgent for not doing so, but the self-indulgent man is so called because he is pained more than he ought at not getting pleasant things (even his pain being caused by pleasure), and the temperate man is so called because he is not pained at the absence of what is pleasant and at his abstinence from it.

The self-indulgent man, then, craves for all pleasant things or those that are most pleasant, and is led by his appetite to choose these at the cost of everything else; hence he is pained both when he fails to get them and when he is merely craving for them (for appetite involves pain); but it seems absurd to be pained for the sake of pleasure. People who fall short with regard to pleasures and delight in them less than they should are hardly found; for such insensibility is not human. Even the other animals distinguish different kinds of food and enjoy some and not others; and if there is anyone who finds nothing pleasant and nothing more attractive than anything else, he must be something quite different from a man; this sort of person has not received a name because he hardly occurs. The temperate man occupies a middle position with regard to these objects. For he neither enjoys the things that the self-indulgent man enjoys most – but rather dislikes them – nor in general the things that he should not, nor anything of this sort to excess, nor does he feel pain or craving when they are absent, or does so only to a moderate degree, and not more than he should, nor when he should not, and so on; but the things that, being pleasant, make for health or for good condition, he will desire moderately and as he should, and also other pleasant things if they are not hindrances to these ends, or contrary to what is noble, or beyond his means. For he who neglects these conditions loves such pleasures more than they are worth, but the temperate man is not that sort of person, but the sort of person that the right rule prescribes.

Self-indulgence more voluntary than cowardice: comparison of the self-indulgent man to the spoilt child

12.   Self-indulgence is more like a voluntary state than cowardice. For the former is actuated by pleasure, the latter by pain, of which the one is to be chosen and the other to be avoided; and pain upsets and destroys the nature of the person who feels it, while pleasure does nothing of the sort. Therefore self-indulgence is more voluntary. Hence also it is more a matter of reproach; for it is easier to become accustomed to its objects, since there are many things of this sort in life, and the process of habituation to them is free from danger, while with terrible objects the reverse is the case. But cowardice would seem to be voluntary in a different degree from its particular manifestations; for it is itself painless, but in these we are upset by pain, so that we even throw down our arms and disgrace ourselves in other ways; hence our acts are even thought to be done under compulsion. For the self-indulgent man, on the other hand, the particular acts are voluntary (for he does them with craving and desire), but the whole state is less so; for no one craves to be self-indulgent.

The name self-indulgence is applied also to childish faults;[21] for they bear a certain resemblance to what we have been considering. Which is called after which, makes no difference to our present purpose; plainly, however, the later is called after the earlier. The transference of the name seems not a bad one; for that which desires what is base and which develops quickly ought to be kept in a chastened condition, and these characteristics belong above all to appetite and to the child, since children in fact live at the beck and call of appetite, and it is in them that the desire for what is pleasant is strongest. If, then, it is not going to be obedient and subject to the ruling principle, it will go to great lengths; for in an irrational being the desire for pleasure is insatiable even if it tries every source of gratification, and the exercise of appetite increases its innate force, and if appetites are strong and violent they even expel the power of calculation. Hence they should be moderate and few, and should in no way oppose the rational principle – and this is what we call an obedient and chastened state – and as the child should live according to the direction of his tutor, so the appetitive element should live according to rational principle. Hence the appetitive element in a temperate man should harmonize with the rational principle; for the noble is the mark at which both aim, and the temperate man craves for the things he ought, as he ought, and when he ought; and this is what rational principle directs.

Here we conclude our account of temperance.

Notes

1   1107^{a}33–^{b}4.
2   1107^{b}2, cf. 1107^{b}29, 1108^{a}5.
3   Ch. 6.

4 1115^{b}11–24.
5 *Il.* xxii. 100.
6 *Il.* viii. 148, 149.
7 Chs. 6, 7.
8 Aristotle's quotation is more like *Il.* ii. 391–3, where Agamemnon speaks, than xv. 348–51, where Hector speaks.
9 The reference is to a battle at Coronea in the Sacred War, *c.* 353 B.C., in which the Phocians defeated the citizens of Coronea and some Boeotian regulars.
10 This is a conflation of *Il.* xi. 11 or xiv. 151 and xvi. 529.
11 Cf. *Il.* v. 470, xv. 232, 594.
12 Cf. *Od.* xxiv. 318f.
13 The phrase does not occur in Homer; it is found in Theocr. xx. 15.
14 1115^{b}11–24.
15 Ibid.
16 At the Long Walls of Corinth, 392 B.C. Cf. Xen. *Hell.* iv. 4. 10.
17 1115^{b}7–13.
18 1107^{b}4–6.
19 *Il.* iii. 24.
20 *Il.* xxiv. 130.
21 ἀκόλαστος, which we have translated 'self-indulgent', meant originally 'unchastened' and was applied to the ways of spoilt children.

Book VI – Intellectual Virtue

Introduction

Reasons for studying intellectual virtue: intellect divided into the contemplative and the calculative

1. Since we have previously said that one ought to choose that which is intermediate, not the excess nor the defect,[1] and that the intermediate is determined by the dictates of the right rule,[2] let us discuss the nature of these dictates. In all the states of character we have mentioned,[3] as in all other matters, there is a mark to which the man who has the rule looks, and heightens or relaxes his activity accordingly, and there is a standard which determines the mean states which we say are intermediate between excess and defect, being in accordance with the right rule. But such a statement, though true, is by no means clear; for not only here but in all other pursuits which are objects of knowledge it is indeed true to say that we must not exert ourselves nor relax our efforts too much or too little, but to an intermediate extent and as the right rule dictates; but if a man had only this knowledge he would be none the wiser – e.g. we should not know what sort of medicines to apply to our body if someone were to say 'all those which the medical art prescribes, and which agree with the practice of one who possesses the art'. Hence it is necessary with regard to the states of the soul also, not only that this true statement should be made, but also that it should be determined what is the right rule and what is the standard that fixes it.

We divided the virtues of the soul and said that some are virtues of character and others of intellect.[4] Now we have discussed in detail the moral virtues;[5] with regard to the others let us express our view as follows, beginning with some remarks about the soul. We said before[6] that there are two parts of the soul – that which grasps a rule or rational principle, and the irrational; let us now draw a similar distinction within the part which grasps a rational principle. And let it be assumed that there are two parts which grasp a rational principle – one by which we contemplate the kind of things whose originative causes are invariable, and one by which we contemplate variable things; for where objects differ in kind the part of the soul answering to each of the two is different in kind, since it is in virtue of a certain likeness and kinship with their objects that they have the knowledge they have. Let one of these parts be called the scientific and the other the calculative; for to deliberate and to calculate are the same thing, but no one deliberates about the invariable. Therefore the calculative is one part of the faculty which grasps a rational principle. We must, then, learn what is the best state of each of these two parts; for this is the virtue of each.

The proper object of contemplation is truth; that of calculation is truth corresponding with right desire

2.   The virtue of a thing is relative to its proper work. Now there are three things in the soul which control action and truth – sensation, reason, desire.

Of these sensation originates no action; this is plain from the fact that the lower animals have sensation but no share in action.

What affirmation and negation are in thinking, pursuit and avoidance are in desire; so that since moral virtue is a state of character concerned with choice, and choice is deliberate desire, therefore both the reasoning must be true and the desire right, if the choice is to be good, and the latter must pursue just what the former asserts. Now this kind of intellect and of truth is practical; of the intellect which is contemplative, not practical nor productive, the good and the bad state are truth and falsity respectively (for this is the work of everything intellectual); while of the part which is practical and intellectual the good state is truth in agreement with right desire.

The origin of action – its efficient, not its final cause – is choice, and that of choice is desire and reasoning with a view to an end. This is why choice cannot exist either without reason and intellect or without a moral state; for good action and its opposite cannot exist without a combination of intellect and character. Intellect itself, however, moves nothing, but only the intellect which aims at an end and is practical; for this rules the productive intellect as well, since everyone who makes makes for an end, and that which is made is not an end in the unqualified sense (but only an end in a particular relation, and the end of a particular operation) – only that which is *done* is that; for good action is an end, and desire aims at this. Hence choice is either desiderative reason or ratiocinative desire, and such an origin of action is a man. (It is to be noted that nothing that is past is an object of choice, e.g. no one chooses to have sacked Troy; for no one *deliberates* about the past, but about what is future and capable of being otherwise, while what is past is not capable of not having taken place; hence Agathon is right in saying:

> For this alone is lacking even to God,
> To make undone things that have once been done.)

The work of both the intellectual parts, then, is truth. Therefore the states that are most strictly those in respect of which each of these parts will reach truth are the virtues of the two parts.

The chief intellectual virtues

Science – demonstrative knowledge of the necessary and eternal

3. Let us begin, then, from the beginning, and discuss these states once more. Let it be assumed that the states by virtue of which the soul possesses truth by way of affirmation or denial are five in number, i.e. art, scientific knowledge, practical wisdom, philosophic wisdom, intuitive reason; we do not include judgement and opinion because in these we may be mistaken.

Now what *scientific knowledge* is, if we are to speak exactly and not follow mere similarities, is plain from what follows. We all suppose that what we know is not even capable of being otherwise; of things capable of being otherwise we do not know, when they have passed outside our observation, whether they exist or not. Therefore the object of scientific knowledge is of necessity. Therefore it is eternal; for things that are of necessity in the unqualified sense are all eternal; and things that are eternal are ungenerated and imperishable. Again, every science is thought to be capable of being taught, and its object of being learnt. And all teaching starts from what is already known, as we maintain in the *Analytics* also; for it proceeds sometimes through induction and sometimes by syllogism. Now induction is the starting-point which knowledge even of the universal presupposes, while syllogism proceeds *from* universals. There are therefore starting-points from which syllogism proceeds, which are not reached by syllogism; it is therefore by induction that they are acquired. Scientific knowledge is, then, a state of capacity to demonstrate, and has the other limiting characteristics which we specify in the *Analytics*; for it is when a man believes in a certain way and the starting-points are known to him that he has scientific knowledge, since if they are not better known to him than the conclusion, he will have his knowledge only incidentally.

Let this, then, be taken as our account of scientific knowledge.

Art – knowledge of how to make things

4.   In the variable are included both things made and things done; making and acting are different (for their nature we treat even the discussions outside our school as reliable); so that the reasoned state of capacity to act is different from the reasoned state of capacity to make. Hence too they are not included one in the other; for neither is acting making nor is making acting. Now since architecture is an art and is essentially a reasoned state of capacity to make, and there is neither any art that is not such a state nor any such state that is not an art, *art* is identical with a state of capacity to make, involving a true course of reasoning. All art is concerned with coming into being, i.e. with contriving and considering how something may come into being which is capable of either being or not being, and whose origin is in the maker and not in the thing made; for art is concerned neither with things that are, or come into being, by necessity, nor with things that do so in accordance with nature (since these have their origin in themselves). Making and acting being different, art must be a matter of making, not of acting. And in a sense chance and art are concerned with the same objects; as Agathon says, 'Art loves chance and chance loves art'. Art, then, as has been said,[7] is a state concerned with making, involving a true course of reasoning, and lack of art on the contrary is a state concerned with making, involving a false course of reasoning; both are concerned with the variable.

Practical wisdom – knowledge of how to secure the ends of human life

5. Regarding *practical wisdom* we shall get at the truth by considering who are the persons we credit with it. Now it is thought to be a mark of a man of practical wisdom to be able to deliberate well about what is good and expedient for himself, not in some particular respect, e.g. about what sorts of thing conduce to health or to strength, but about what sorts of thing conduce to the good life in general. This is shown by the fact that we credit men with practical wisdom in some particular respect when they have calculated well with a view to some good end which is one of those that are not the object of any art. It follows that in the general sense also the man who is capable of deliberating has practical wisdom. Now no one deliberates about things that are invariable, or about things that it is impossible for him to do. Therefore, since scientific knowledge involves demonstration, but there is no demonstration of things whose first principles are variable (for all such things might actually be otherwise), and since it is impossible to deliberate about things that are of necessity, practical wisdom cannot be scientific knowledge or art; not science because that which can be done is capable of being otherwise, not art because action and making are different kinds of thing. The remaining alternative, then, is that it is a true and reasoned state of capacity to act with regard to the things that are good or bad for man. For while making has an end other than itself, action cannot; for good action itself is its end. It is for this reason that we think Pericles and men like him have practical wisdom, viz. because they can see what is good for themselves and what is good for men in general; we consider that those can do this who are good at managing households or states. (This is why we call temperance (*sōphrosunē*) by this name; we imply that it preserves one's practical wisdom (*sōzousa tēn phronēsin*). Now what it preserves is a judgement of the kind we have described. For it is not any and every judgement that pleasant and painful objects destroy and pervert, e.g. the judgement that the triangle has or has not its angles equal to two right angles, but only judgements about what is to be done. For the originating causes of the things that are done consist in the end at which they are aimed; but the man who has been ruined by pleasure or pain forthwith fails to see any such originating cause – to see that for the sake of this or because of this he ought to choose and do whatever he chooses and does; for vice is destructive of the originating cause of action.)

Practical wisdom, then, must be a reasoned and true state of capacity to act with regard to human goods. But further, while there is such a thing as excellence in art, there is no such thing as excellence in practical wisdom; and in art he who errs willingly is preferable, but in practical wisdom, as in the virtues, he is the reverse. Plainly, then, practical wisdom is a virtue and not an art. There being two parts of the soul that can follow a course of reasoning, it must be a virtue of one of the two, i.e. of that part which forms opinions; for opinion is about the variable and so is practical wisdom. But yet it is not only a reasoned state; this is shown by the fact that a state of that sort may be forgotten but practical wisdom cannot.

Intuitive reason – knowledge of the principles from which science proceeds

6.   Scientific knowledge is judgement about things that are universal and necessary; and the conclusions of demonstration, and all scientific knowledge, follow from first principles (for scientific knowledge involves proof). This being so, the first principle from which what is scientifically known follows cannot be an object of scientific knowledge, of art, or of practical wisdom; for that which can be scientifically known can be demonstrated, and art and practical wisdom deal with things that are variable. Nor are these first principles the objects of philosophic wisdom, for it is a mark of the philosopher to have *demonstration* about some things. If, then, the states of mind by which we have truth and are never deceived about things invariable or even variable are scientific knowledge, practical wisdom, philosophic wisdom, and intuitive reason, and it cannot be any of the three (i.e. practical wisdom, scientific knowledge, or philosophic wisdom), the remaining alternative is that it is *intuitive reason* that grasps the first principles.

Philosophic wisdom – the union of intuitive reason and science

7.   *Wisdom*[8] (1) in the arts we ascribe to their most finished exponents, e.g. to Phidias as a sculptor and to Polyclitus as a maker of portrait-statues, and here we mean nothing by wisdom except excellence in art; but (2) we think that some people are wise in general, not in some particular field or in any other limited respect, as Homer says in the *Margites*,

> Him did the gods make neither a digger nor yet
> a ploughman
> Nor wise in anything else.

Therefore wisdom must plainly be the most finished of the forms of knowledge. It follows that the wise man must not only know what follows from the first principles, but must also possess truth about the first principles. Therefore wisdom must be intuitive reason combined with scientific knowledge – scientific knowledge of the highest objects which has received as it were its proper completion.

Of the highest objects, we say; for it would be strange to think that the art of politics, or practical wisdom, is the best knowledge, since man is not the best thing in the world. Now if what is healthy or good is different for men and for fishes, but what is white or straight is always the same, anyone would say that what is wise is the same but what is practically wise is different; for it is to that which considers well the various matters concerning itself that one ascribes practical wisdom, and it is to this that one will entrust such matters. This is why we say that some even of the lower animals have practical wisdom,[9] viz. those which are found to have a power of foresight with regard to their own life. It is evident also that philosophic wisdom and the art of politics cannot be the same; for if the state of mind concerned with a man's own interests is to be called philosophic wisdom, there will be many philosophic wisdoms; there will not be one concerned with the good of all animals (any more than there is one art of medicine for all existing things), but a different philosophic wisdom about the good of each species.

But if the argument be that man is the best of the animals, this makes no difference; for there are other things much more divine in their nature even than man, e.g., most conspicuously, the bodies of which the heavens are framed. From what has been said it is plain, then, that philosophic wisdom is scientific knowledge, combined with intuitive reason, of the things that are highest by nature. This is why we say Anaxagoras, Thales, and men like them have philosophic but not practical wisdom, when we see them ignorant of what is to their own advantage, and why we say that they know things that are remarkable, admirable, difficult, and divine, but useless; viz. because it is not human goods that they seek.

Practical wisdom on the other hand is concerned with things human and things about which it is possible to deliberate; for we say this is above all the work of the man of practical wisdom, to deliberate well, but no one deliberates about things invariable, or about things which have not an end which is a good that can be brought about by action. The man who is without qualification good at deliberating is the man who is capable of aiming in accordance with calculation at the best for man of things attainable by action. Nor is practical wisdom concerned with universals only – it must also recognize the particulars; for it is practical, and practice is concerned with particulars. This is why some who do not know, and especially those who have experience, are more practical than others who know; for if a man knew that light meats are digestible and wholesome, but did not know which sorts of meat are light, he would not produce health, but the man who knows that chicken is wholesome is more likely to produce health.

Now practical wisdom is concerned with action; therefore one should have both forms of it, or the latter in preference to the former. But here, too, there must be a controlling kind.

Relations between practical wisdom and political science

8.   Political wisdom and practical wisdom are the same state of mind, but their essence is not the same. Of the wisdom concerned with the city, the practical wisdom which plays a controlling part is legislative wisdom, while that which is related to this as particulars to their universal is known by the general name 'political wisdom'; this has to do with action and deliberation, for a decree is a thing to be carried out in the form of an individual act. This is why the exponents of this art are alone said to 'take part in politics'; for these alone 'do things' as manual labourers 'do things'.

Practical wisdom also is identified especially with that form of it which is concerned with a man himself – with the individual; and this is known by the general name 'practical wisdom'; of the other kinds one is called household management, another legislation, the third politics, and of the latter one part is called deliberative and the other judicial. Now knowing what is good for oneself will be one kind of knowledge, but it is very different from the other kinds; and the man who knows and concerns himself with his own interests is thought to have practical wisdom, while politicians are thought to be busybodies; hence the words of Euripides:

> But how could I be wise, who might at ease,
> Numbered among the army's multitude,
> Have had an equal share? . . .
> For those who aim too high and do too much. . . .

Those who think thus seek their own good, and consider that one ought to do so. From this opinion, then, has come the view that such men have practical wisdom; yet perhaps one's own good cannot exist without household management, nor without a form of government. Further, how one should order one's own affairs is not clear and needs inquiry.

What has been said is confirmed by the fact that while young men become geometricians and mathematicians and wise in matters like these, it is thought that a young man of practical wisdom cannot be found. The cause is that such wisdom is concerned not only with universals but with particulars, which become familiar from experience, but a young man has no experience, for it is length of time that gives experience; indeed one might ask this question too, why a boy may become a mathematician, but not a philosopher or a physicist. Is it because the objects of mathematics exist by abstraction, while the first principles of these other subjects come from experience, and because young men have no conviction about the latter but merely use the proper language, while the essence of mathematical objects is plain enough to them?

Further, error in deliberation may be either about the universal or about the particular; we may fail to know either that all water that weighs heavy is bad, or that this particular water weighs heavy.

That practical wisdom is not scientific knowledge is evident; for it is, as has been said,[10] concerned with the ultimate particular fact, since the thing to be done is of this nature. It is opposed, then, to intuitive reason; for intuitive reason is of the limiting premises, for which no reason can be given, while practical wisdom is concerned with the ultimate particular, which is the object not of scientific knowledge but of perception – not the perception of qualities peculiar to one sense but a perception akin to that by which we perceive that the particular figure before us is a triangle; for in that direction as well there will be a limit. But this is rather perception than practical wisdom, though it is another kind of perception than that of the qualities peculiar to each sense.

Minor intellectual virtues concerned with conduct

Goodness in deliberation, how related to practical wisdom

9. There is a difference between inquiry and deliberation; for deliberation is a particular kind of inquiry. We must grasp the nature of excellence in deliberation as well – whether it is a form of scientific knowledge, or opinion, or skill in conjecture, or some other kind of thing. *Scientific knowledge* it is not; for men do not inquire about the things they know about, but good deliberation is a kind of deliberation, and he who deliberates inquires and calculates. Nor is it *skill in conjecture*; for this both involves no reasoning and is something that is quick in its operation, while men deliberate a long time, and they say that one should carry out quickly the conclusions of one's deliberation, but should deliberate slowly. Again, *readiness of mind* is different from excellence in deliberation; it is a sort of skill in conjecture. Nor again is excellence in deliberation *opinion* of any sort. But since the man who deliberates badly makes a mistake, while he who deliberates well does so correctly, excellence in deliberation is clearly a kind of correctness, but neither of knowledge nor of opinion; for there is no such thing as correctness of knowledge (since there is no such thing as error of knowledge), and correctness of opinion is truth; and at the same time everything that is an object of opinion is already determined. But again excellence in deliberation involves reasoning. The remaining alternative, then, is that it is *correctness of thinking*; for this is not yet assertion, since, while even opinion is not inquiry but has reached the stage of assertion, the man who is deliberating, whether he does so well or ill, is searching for something and calculating.

But excellence in deliberation is a certain correctness of deliberation; hence we must first inquire what deliberation is and what it is about. And, there being more than one kind of correctness, plainly excellence in deliberation is not any and every kind; for (1) the incontinent man and the bad man, if he is clever, will reach as a result of his calculation what he sets before himself, so that he will have deliberated correctly, but he will have got for himself a great evil. Now to have deliberated well is thought to be a good thing; for it is this kind of correctness of deliberation that is excellence in deliberation, viz. that which tends to attain what is good. But (2) it is possible to attain even good by a false syllogism, and to attain what one ought to do but not by the right means, the middle term being false; so that this too is not yet excellence in deliberation – this state in virtue of which one attains what one ought but not by the right means. Again (3) it is possible to attain it by long deliberation while another man attains it quickly. Therefore in the former case we have not yet got excellence in deliberation, which is rightness with regard to the expedient – rightness in respect both of the end, the manner, and the time. (4) Further, it is possible to have deliberated well either in the unqualified sense or with reference to a particular end. Excellence in deliberation in the unqualified sense, then, is that which succeeds with reference to what is the end in the unqualified sense, and excellence in deliberation in a particular sense is that which succeeds relatively to a particular end. If, then, it is characteristic of men of practical wisdom to have deliberated well, excellence in deliberation will be correctness with regard to what conduces to the end which practical wisdom apprehends truly.

Understanding – the critical quality answering to the imperative quality practical wisdom

10.   Understanding, also, and goodness of understanding, in virtue of which men are said to be men of understanding or of good understanding, are neither entirely the same as opinion or scientific knowledge (for at that rate all men would have been men of understanding), nor are they one of the particular sciences, such as medicine, the science of things connected with health, or geometry, the science of spatial magnitudes. For understanding is neither about things that are always and are unchangeable, nor about any and every one of the things that come into being, but about things which may become subjects of questioning and deliberation. Hence it is about the same objects as practical wisdom; but understanding and practical wisdom are not the same. For practical wisdom issues commands, since its end is what ought to be done or not to be done; but understanding only judges. (Understanding is identical with goodness of understanding, men of understanding with men of good understanding.) Now understanding is neither the having nor the acquiring of practical wisdom; but as learning is called understanding when it means the exercise of the faculty of knowledge,[11] so 'understanding' is applicable to the exercise of the faculty of opinion for the purpose of judging of what someone else says about matters with which practical wisdom is concerned – and of judging soundly; for 'well' and 'soundly' are the same thing. And from this has come the use of the name 'understanding' in virtue of which men are said to be 'of good understanding', viz. from the application of the word to the grasping of scientific truth; for we often call such grasping understanding.

Judgement – right discrimination of the equitable: the place of intuition in morals

11.   What is called judgement, in virtue of which men are said to 'be sympathetic judges' and to 'have judgement', is the right discrimination of the equitable. This is shown by the fact that we say the equitable man is above all others a man of sympathetic judgement, and identify equity with sympathetic judgement about certain facts. And sympathetic judgement is judgement which discriminates what is equitable and does so correctly; and correct judgement is that which judges what is true.

Now all the states we have considered converge, as might be expected, to the same point; for when we speak of judgement and understanding and practical wisdom and intuitive reason we credit the same people with possessing judgement and having reached years of reason and with having practical wisdom and understanding. For all these faculties deal with ultimates, i.e. with particulars; and being a man of understanding and of good or sympathetic judgement consists in being able to judge about the things with which practical wisdom is concerned; for the equities are common to all good men in relation to other men. Now all things which have to be done are included among particulars or ultimates; for not only must the man of practical wisdom know particular facts, but understanding and judgement are also concerned with things to be done, and these are ultimates. And intuitive reason is concerned with the ultimates in both directions; for both the first terms and the last are objects of intuitive reason and not of argument, and the intuitive reason which is presupposed by demonstrations grasps the unchangeable and first terms, while the intuitive reason involved in practical reasonings grasps the last and variable fact, i.e. the minor premiss. For these variable facts are the starting-points for the apprehension of the end, since the universals are reached from the particulars; of these therefore we must have perception, and this perception is intuitive reason.

This is why these states are thought to be natural endowments – why, while no one is thought to be a philosopher by nature, people are thought to have by nature judgement, understanding, and intuitive reason. This is shown by the fact that we think our powers correspond to our time of life, and that a particular age brings with it intuitive reason and judgement; this implies that nature is the cause. [Hence intuitive reason is both beginning and end; for demonstrations are from these and about these.[12]] Therefore we ought to attend to the undemonstrated sayings and opinions of experienced and older people or of people of practical wisdom not less than to demonstrations; for because experience has given them an eye they see aright.

We have stated, then, what practical and philosophic wisdom are, and with what each of them is concerned, and we have said that each is the virtue of a different part of the soul.

Relation of philosophic to practical wisdom

What is the use of philosophic and of practical wisdom? Philosophic wisdom is the formal cause of happiness; practical wisdom is what ensures the taking of proper means to the proper ends desired by moral virtue

12.   Difficulties might be raised as to the utility of these qualities of mind. For (1) philosophic wisdom will contemplate none of the things that will make a man happy (for it is not concerned with any coming into being), and though practical wisdom has *this* merit, for what purpose do we need it? Practical wisdom is the quality of mind concerned with things just and noble and good for man, but these are the things which it is the mark of a *good* man to do, and we are none the more able to act for *knowing* them if the virtues are states of *character*, just as we are none the better able to act for knowing the things that are healthy and sound, in the sense not of producing but of issuing from the state of health; for we are none the more able to act for having the art of medicine or of gymnastics. But (2) if we are to say that a man should have practical wisdom not for the sake of knowing moral truths but for the sake of becoming good, practical wisdom will be of no use to those who *are* good; but again it is of no use to those who have *not* virtue; for it will make no difference whether they have practical wisdom themselves or obey others who have it, and it would be enough for us to do what we do in the case of health; though we wish to become healthy, yet we do not learn the art of medicine. (3) Besides this, it would be thought strange if practical wisdom, being inferior to philosophic wisdom, is to be put in authority over it, as seems to be implied by the fact that the art which produces anything rules and issues commands about that thing.

These, then, are the questions we must discuss; so far we have only stated the difficulties.

(1)   Now first let us say that in themselves these states must be worthy of choice because they are the virtues of the two parts of the soul respectively, even if neither of them produces anything.

(2)   Secondly, they do produce something, not as the art of medicine produces health, however, but as health produces health;[13] so does philosophic wisdom produce happiness; for, being a part of virtue entire, by being possessed and by actualizing itself it makes a man happy.

(3)   Again, the work of man is achieved only in accordance with practical wisdom as well as with moral virtue; for virtue makes us aim at the right mark, and practical wisdom makes us take the right means. (Of the fourth part of the soul – the nutritive[14] – there is no such virtue; for there is nothing which it is in its power to do or not to do.)

(4)   With regard to our being none the more able to do because of our practical wisdom what is noble and just, let us begin a little further back, starting with the following principle. As we say that some people who do just acts are not necessarily just, i.e. those who do the acts ordained by the laws either unwillingly or owing to ignorance or for some other reason and not for the sake of the acts themselves (though, to be sure, they do what they should and all the things that the good man ought), so is it, it seems, that in order to be good one must be in a certain state when one does the several acts, i.e. one must do them as a result of choice and for the sake of the acts themselves. Now virtue makes the choice right, but the question of the things which should naturally be done to carry out

our choice belongs not to virtue but to another faculty. We must devote our attention to these matters and give a clearer statement about them. There is a faculty which is called cleverness; and this is such as to be able to do the things that tend towards the mark we have set before ourselves, and to hit it. Now if the mark be noble, the cleverness is laudable, but if the mark be bad, the cleverness is mere smartness; hence we call even men of practical wisdom clever or smart. Practical wisdom is not the faculty, but it does not exist without this faculty. And this eye of the soul acquires its formed state not without the aid of virtue, as has been said[15] and is plain; for the syllogisms which deal with acts to be done are things which involve a starting-point, viz. 'since the end, i.e. what is best, is of such and such a nature', whatever it may be (let it for the sake of argument be what we please); and this is not evident except to the good man; for wickedness perverts us and causes us to be deceived about the starting-points of action. Therefore it is evident that it is impossible to be practically wise without being good.

Relation of practical wisdom to natural virtue, moral virtue, and the right rule

13.   We must therefore consider virtue also once more; for virtue too is similarly related; as practical wisdom is to cleverness – not the same, but like it – so is natural virtue to virtue in the strict sense. For all men think that each type of character belongs to its possessors in some sense by nature; for from the very moment of birth we are just or fitted for self-control or brave or have the other moral qualities; but yet we seek something else as that which is good in the strict sense – we seek for the presence of such qualities in another way. For both children and brutes have the natural dispositions to these qualities, but without reason these are evidently hurtful. Only we seem to see this much, that, while one may be led astray by them, as a strong body which moves without sight may stumble badly because of its lack of sight, still, if a man once acquires reason, that makes a difference in action; and his state, while still like what it was, will then be virtue in the strict sense. Therefore, as in the part of us which forms opinions there are two types, cleverness and practical wisdom, so too in the moral part there are two types, natural virtue and virtue in the strict sense, and of these the latter involves practical wisdom. This is why some say that all the virtues are forms of practical wisdom, and why Socrates in one respect was on the right track while in another he went astray; in thinking that all the virtues were forms of practical wisdom he was wrong, but in saying they implied practical wisdom he was right. This is confirmed by the fact that even now all men, when they define virtue, after naming the state of character and its objects add 'that (state) which is in accordance with the right rule'; now the right rule is that which is in accordance with practical wisdom. All men, then, seem somehow to divine that this kind of state is virtue, viz. that which is in accordance with practical wisdom. But we must go a little further. For it is not merely the state in accordance with the right rule, but the state that implies the *presence* of the right rule, that is virtue; and practical wisdom is a right rule about such matters. Socrates, then, thought the virtues were rules or rational principles (for he thought they were, all of them, forms of scientific knowledge), while we think they *involve* a rational principle.

It is clear, then, from what has been said, that it is not possible to be good in the strict sense without practical wisdom, or practically wise without moral virtue. But in this way we may also refute the dialectical argument whereby it might be contended that the virtues exist in separation from each other; the same man, it might be said, is not best equipped by nature for all the virtues, so that he will have already acquired one when he has not yet acquired another. This is possible in respect of the natural virtues, but not in respect of those in respect of which a man is called without qualification good; for with the presence of the one quality, practical wisdom, will be given all the virtues. And it is plain that, even if it were of no practical value, we should have needed it because it is the virtue of the part of us in question; plain too that the choice will not be right without practical wisdom any more than without virtue; for the one determines the end and the other makes us do the things that lead to the end.

But again it is not *supreme* over philosophic wisdom, i.e. over the superior part of us, any more than the art of medicine is over health; for it does not use it but provides for its coming into being; it issues orders, then, for its sake, but not to it. Further, to maintain its supremacy would be like saying that the art of politics rules the gods because it issues orders about all the affairs of the state.

Notes

1 1104ᵃ11–27, 1106ᵃ26–1107ᵃ27.
2 1107ᵃ1, cf. 1103ᵇ31, 1114ᵇ29.
3 In iii. 6–v. 11.
4 1103ᵃ3–7.
5 In iii. 6–v. 11.
6 1102ᵃ26–28.

7 l. 9.

8 In this chapter Aristotle restricts to a very definite meaning the word σοφία, which in ordinary Greek, as the beginning of the chapter points out, was used both of skill in a particular art or craft, and of wisdom in general.

9 We do not say this in English; but we call them 'intelligent' or 'sagacious', which comes to the same thing.

10 1141^{b}14–22.

11 This is a use of μανθάνειν which is not shared by its normal English equivalent, 'learn'.

12 This sentence should probably be read, as Bywater suggests, at the end of the previous paragraph.

13 i.e. as health, as an inner state, produces the activities which we know as constituting health.

14 The other three being the scientific (τὸ ἐπιστημονικόν), the calculative (τὸ λογιστικόν), and the desiderative (τὸ ὀρεκτικόν).

15 ll. 6–26.

2

From *An Inquiry into the Original of Our Idea of Virtue*

Francis Hutcheson

Introduction

The word *moral goodness*, in this treatise, denotes our idea of some quality apprehended in actions, which procures approbation attended with desire of the agent's happiness. *Moral evil* denotes our idea of a contrary quality, which excites condemnation or dislike. Approbation and condemnation are probably simple ideas, which cannot be farther explained. We must be contented with these imperfect descriptions, until we discover whether we really have such ideas, and what general foundation there is in nature for this difference of actions, as morally good or evil.

These descriptions seem to contain an universally acknowledged difference of *moral good* and *evil*, from *natural*. All men who speak of moral good, acknowledge that it procures approbation and good-will toward those we apprehend possessed of it; whereas natural good does not. In this matter men must consult their own breasts. How differently are they affected toward these they suppose possessed of honesty, faith, generosity, kindness; and those who are possessed of the natural goods, such as houses, lands, gardens, vineyards, health, strength, sagacity? We shall find that we necessarily love and approve the possessors of the former; but the possession of the latter procures no approbation or good-will at all toward the possessor, but often contrary affections of envy and hatred. In the same manner, whatever quality we apprehend to be morally evil, raises

Francis Hutcheson, *Philosophical Writings* (London: J. M. Dent, 1994), pp. 67–8, 70–3, 75–7, 80–4.

our dislike toward the person in whom we observe it, such as treachery, cruelty, ingratitude; whereas we heartily love, esteem, and pity many who are exposed to natural evils, such as pain, poverty, hunger, sickness, death.

Now the first question on this subject is, 'Whence arise these different ideas of actions?'

Because we shall afterwards frequently use the words *interest*, *advantage, natural good*, it is necessary here to fix their ideas. The pleasure in our sensible perceptions of any kind, gives us our first idea of *natural good* or *happiness*; and then all objects which are apt to excite this pleasure are called *immediately good*. Those objects which may procure others immediately pleasant, are called *advantageous*; and we pursue both kinds from a view of *interest*, or from *self-love*.

Our *sense* of pleasure is antecedent to advantage or interest, and is the foundation of it. We do not perceive pleasure in objects, because it is our interest to do so; but objects or actions are advantageous, and are pursued or undertaken from interest, because we receive pleasure from them. Our perception of pleasure is necessary, and nothing is advantageous or naturally good to us, but what is apt to raise pleasure mediately, or immediately. Such objects as we know either from experience of sense, or reason, to be immediately or mediately advantageous, or apt to minister pleasure, we are said to pursue from *self-interest*, when our intention is only to enjoy this pleasure, which they have the power of exciting. Thus meats, drink, harmony, fine prospects, painting, statues, are perceived by our senses to be immediately good; and our reason shows riches and power to be mediately so, that is, apt to furnish us with objects of immediate pleasure: and both kinds of these natural goods are pursued from interest, or self-love.

Section I:
Of the Moral Sense by which we perceive Virtue and Vice, and approve or disapprove them in others

I.   That the perceptions of *moral good* and *evil*, are perfectly different from those of *natural good* or *advantage*, every one must convince himself, by reflecting upon the different manner in which he finds himself affected when these objects occur to him. Had we no sense of good distinct from the advantage or interest arising from the external senses, and the perceptions of beauty and harmony; the sensations and affections toward a fruitful field, or commodious habitation, would be much the same with what we have toward a generous friend, or any noble character; for both are or may be advantageous to us: and we should no more admire any action, or love any person in a distant country, or age, whose influence could not extend to us, than we love the mountains of Peru, while we are unconcerned in the Spanish trade. We should have the same sentiments and affections toward inanimate beings, which we have toward rational agents, which yet everyone knows to be false. Upon comparison, we say, 'Why should we approve or love inanimate beings? They have no intention of good to us, or to any other person; their nature makes them fit for our uses, which they neither know nor study to serve. But it is not so with rational agents: they study the interest, and desire the happiness of other beings with whom they converse.'

We are all then conscious of the difference between that *approbation* or perception of *moral excellence*, which *benevolence* excites toward the person in whom we observe it, and that opinion of *natural goodness*, which only raises *desire* of possession toward the good object. Now 'what should make this difference, if all approbation, or sense of good be from prospect of advantage? Do not inanimate objects promote our advantage as well as benevolent persons, who do us offices of kindness and friendship? should we not then have the same endearing approbation of both? or only the same cold opinion of advantage in both?' The reason why it is not so, must be this, 'that we have a distinct perception of *beauty* or *excellence* in the kind affections of rational agents; whence we are determined to admire and love such characters and persons.'

Suppose we reap the same advantage from two men, one of whom serves us from an ultimate desire of our happiness, or good-will toward us; the other from views of self-interest, or by constraint: both are in this case equally beneficial or advantageous to us, and yet we shall have quite different sentiments of them. We must then certainly have other perceptions of moral actions, than those of advantage: and that power of receiving these perceptions may be called a *moral sense*, since the definition agrees to it, viz. a determination of the mind, to receive any idea from the presence of an object which occurs to us, independent on our will.

This perhaps will be equally evident from our ideas of evil, done to us designedly by a rational agent. Our senses of natural good and evil would make us receive, with equal serenity and composure, an assault, a buffet, an affront from a neighbour, a cheat from a partner, or trustee, as we would an equal damage from the fall of a beam, a tile, or a tempest; and we should have the same affections and sentiments on both occasions. Villainy, treachery, cruelty, would be as meekly resented as a blast, or mildew, or an overflowing stream. But I fancy every one is very differently affected on these occasions, though there may be equal natural evil in both. Nay, actions no way detrimental may occasion the strongest anger and indignation, if they evidence only impotent hatred or contempt. And, on the other hand, the intervention of moral ideas may prevent our condemnation of the agent, or bad moral apprehension of that action, which causes to us the greatest natural evil. Thus the opinion of justice in any sentence, will prevent all ideas of moral evil in the execution, or hatred toward the magistrate, who is the immediate cause of our greatest sufferings.

II.   In our sentiments of actions which affect ourselves, there is indeed a mixture of the ideas of natural and moral good, which require some attention to separate them. But when we reflect upon the actions which affect other persons only, we may observe the moral ideas unmixed with those of natural good or evil. For let it be here observed, that those senses by which we perceive pleasure in natural objects, whence they are constituted advantageous, could never raise in us any desire of *public good*, but only of what was good to ourselves in particular. Nor could they ever make us approve an action merely because of its promoting the happiness of others. And yet, as soon as any action is represented to us as flowing from love, humanity, gratitude, compassion, a study of the good of others, and an ultimate desire of their happiness, although it were in the most distant part of the world, or in some past age, we feel joy within us, admire the lovely action, and praise its author. And on the contrary, every action represented as flowing from ill-will, desire of the misery of others without view to any prevalent good to the public, or ingratitude, raises abhorrence and aversion.

It is true indeed, that the actions we approve in others, are generally imagined to tend to the natural good of mankind, or of some parts of it. But whence this secret chain between each person and mankind? How is my interest connected with the most distant parts of it? And yet I must admire actions which show good-will toward them, and love the author. Whence this love, compassion, indignation and hatred toward even feigned characters, in the most distant ages, and nations, according as they appear kind, faithful, compassionate, or of the opposite dispositions, toward their imaginary contemporaries? If there is no moral sense, which makes benevolent actions appear beautiful; if all approbation be from the interest of the approver,

What's Hecuba to us, or we to Hecuba?[1]

III.   Some refined explainers of self-love may tell us, 'that we approve or condemn characters, according as we apprehend we should have been supported, or injured by them, had we lived in their days.' But how obvious is the answer, if we only observe, that had we no sense of moral good in humanity, mercy, faithfulness, why should not self-love, and our sense of natural good engage us always to the victorious side, and make us admire and love the successful tyrant, or traitor? Why do not we love Sinon or Pyrrhus, in the Aeneid? for, had we been Greeks, these two would have been very advantageous characters. Why are we affected with the fortunes of Priamus, Polites, Choroeubs or Aeneas? Would not the parsimony of a miser be as advantageous to his heir, as the generosity of a worthy man is to his friend? And cannot we as easily imagine ourselves heirs to misers, as the favourites of heroes? Why don't we then approve both alike? It is plain we have some secret sense which determines our approbation without regard to self-interest; otherwise we should always favour the fortunate side without regard to virtue, and suppose ourselves engaged with that party.

As Mr Hobbes explains all the sensations of pity by our fear of the like evils, when by imagination we place ourselves in the case of the sufferers,[2] so others explain all approbation and condemnation of actions in distant ages or nations, by a like effort of imagination: we place ourselves in the case of others, and then discern an imaginary private advantage or disadvantage in these actions. But as his account of pity will never explain how the sensation increases, according to the apprehended worth of the sufferer, or according to the affection we formerly had to him; since the sufferings of any stranger may suggest the same possibility of our suffering the like: so this explication will never account for our high approbation of brave unsuccessful attempts, which we see prove detrimental both to the agent, and to those for whose service they were intended; here there is no private advantage to be imagined. Nor will it account for our abhorrence of such injuries as we are incapable of suffering. Sure, when a man abhors the attempts of the young Tarquin, he does not imagine that he has changed his sex like Caeneus. And then, when one corrects his imagination, by remembering his own situation, and circumstances, we find the moral approbation and condemnation continues as lively as it was before, though the imagination of advantage is gone.

Section I: paragraphs VII–VIII

VII.   If what is said makes it appear, that we have some other amiable idea of actions than that of advantageous to ourselves, we may conclude, 'that this perception of moral good is not derived from custom, education, example, or study.' These give us no new ideas: they might make us see private advantage in actions whose usefulness did not at first appear; or give us opinions of some tendency of actions to our detriment, by some nice deductions of reason, or by a rash prejudice, when upon the first view of the action we should have observed no such thing: but they never could have made us apprehend actions as amiable or odious, without any consideration of our own advantage.

VIII.   It remains then, 'that as the Author of nature has determined us to receive, by our external senses, pleasant or disagreeable ideas of objects, according as they are useful or hurtful to our bodies; and to receive from uniform objects the pleasures of beauty and harmony, to excite us to the pursuit of knowledge, and to reward us for it; or to be an argument to us of his goodness, as the uniformity itself proves his existence, whether we had a sense of beauty in uniformity or not; in the same manner he has given us a *moral sense*, to direct our actions, and to give us still nobler pleasures: so that while we are only intending the good of others, we undesignedly promote our own greatest private good.'

We are not to imagine, that this moral sense, more than the other senses, supposes any innate ideas, knowledge, or practical proposition: we mean by it only a determination of our minds to receive the simple ideas of approbation or condemnation, from actions observed, antecedent to any opinions of advantage or loss to redound to ourselves from them; even as we are pleased with a regular form, or an harmonious composition, without having any knowledge of mathematics, or seeing any advantage in that form or composition, different from the immediate pleasure.

That we may discern more distinctly the difference between moral perceptions and others, let us consider, when we taste a pleasant fruit, we are conscious of pleasure; when another tastes it, we only conclude or form an opinion that he enjoys pleasure; and, abstracting from some previous good-will or anger, his enjoying this pleasure is to us a matter wholly indifferent, raising no new sentiment or affection. But when we are under the influence of a virtuous temper, and thereby engaged in virtuous actions, we are not always conscious of any pleasure, nor are we only pursuing private pleasures, as will appear hereafter: it is only by *reflex acts* upon our temper and conduct, that virtue never fails to give pleasure. When also we judge the temper of another to be virtuous, we do not necessarily imagine him *then* to enjoy pleasure, though we know *reflection* will give it to him: and farther, our apprehension of his virtuous temper raises sentiments of approbation, esteem or admiration, and the affection of good-will toward him. The quality approved by our moral sense is conceived to reside in the person approved, and to be a perfection and dignity in him: approbation of another's virtue is not conceived as making the approver happy, or virtuous, or worthy, though it is attended with some small pleasure. Virtue is then called *amiable* or *lovely*, from its raising good-will or love in spectators toward the agent; and not from the agent's perceiving the virtuous temper to be advantageous to him, or desiring to obtain it under that view. A virtuous temper is called *good* or *beatific*, not that it is always attended with pleasure in the agent; much less that some small pleasure attends the contemplation of it in the approver: but from this, that every spectator is persuaded that the reflex acts of the virtuous agent upon his own temper will give him the highest pleasures. The admired quality is conceived as the perfection of the agent, and such a one as is distinct from the pleasure either in the agent or the approver; though it is a sure source of pleasure to the agent. The perception of the approver, though attended with pleasure, plainly represents something quite distinct from this pleasure; even as the perception of external forms is attended with pleasure, and yet represents something distinct from this pleasure. This may prevent many cavils upon this subject.

Section II:
Concerning the Immediate Motive to Virtuous Actions

The *motives* of human actions, or their immediate causes, would be best understood after considering the passions and affections; but here we shall only consider the springs of the actions which we call *virtuous*, as far as it is necessary to settle the general foundation of the moral sense.

I. Every action, which we apprehend as either *morally good* or *evil*, is always supposed to flow from some *affection* toward sensitive natures; and whatever we call *virtue* or *vice*, is either some such *affection*, or some *action* consequent upon it. Or it may perhaps be enough to make an action or omission, appear vicious, if it argues the want of such affection toward rational agents, as we expect in characters counted morally good. All the actions counted *religious* in any country, are supposed, by those who count them so, to flow from some affections toward the Deity; and whatever we call *social virtue*, we still suppose to flow from affections toward our fellow-creatures: for in this all seem to agree, 'that the external motions, when accompanied with no affections toward God or man, or evidencing no want of the *expected* affections toward either, can have no moral good or evil in them.'

Ask, for instance, the most abstemious hermit, if *temperance* of itself would be morally good, supposing it showed no obedience toward the

Deity, made us no fitter for devotion, or the service of mankind, or the search after truth, than *luxury*; and he will easily grant, that it would be no moral good, though still it might be naturally good or advantageous to health: and mere *courage* or contempt of danger, if we conceive it to have no regard to the defence of the innocent, or repairing of wrongs or self-interst, would only entitle its possessor to bedlam. When such sort of courage is sometimes admired, it is upon some secret apprehension of a good intention in the use of it, or as a natural ability capable of an useful application. *Prudence*, if it was only employed in promoting private interest, is never imagined to be a *virtue*: and *justice*, or observing a strict equality, if it has no regard to the good of mankind, the preservation of rights, and securing peace, is a quality properer for its ordinary *gestamen*, a beam and scales, than for a rational agent. So that these four qualities, commonly called *cardinal virtues*, obtain that name, because they are dispositions universally necessary to promote *public good*, and denote *affections* toward *rational agents*; otherwise there would appear no *virtue* in them.

IV.   There are two ways in which some may deduce benevolence from self-love, the one supposing that 'we voluntarily bring this affection upon ourselves, whenever we have an opinion that it will be for our interest to have this affection, either as it may be immediately pleasant, or may afford pleasant reflection afterwards by our moral sense, or as it may tend to procure some external reward from God or man.' The other scheme alleges no such power in us of raising desire or affection of any kind by our choice or volition; but 'supposes our minds determined by the frame of their nature to desire whatever is apprehended as the means of any private happiness; and that the observation of the happiness of other persons, in many cases is made the necessary occasion of pleasure to the observer, as their misery is the occasion of his uneasiness: and in consequence of this connection, as soon as we have observed it, we begin to desire the happiness of others as the means of obtaining this happiness to ourselves, which we expect from the contemplation of others in a happy state. They allege it to be impossible to desire either the happiness of another, or any event whatsoever, without conceiving it as the means of some happiness or pleasure to ourselves; but own at the same time, that desire is not raised in us directly by any volition, but arises necessarily upon our apprehending any object or event to be conducive to our happiness.'

That the former scheme is not just, may appear from this general consideration, that 'neither benevolence nor any other affection or desire can be directly raised by volition.' If they could, then we could be bribed into any affection whatsoever toward any object, even the most improper: we might raise jealousy, fear, anger, love, toward any sort of persons indifferently by an hire, even as we engage men to external actions, or to the dissimulation of passions; but this every person will by his own reflection find to be impossible. The prospect of any advantage to arise to us from having any affection, may indeed turn our attention to those qualities in the object, which are naturally constituted the necessary causes or occasions of the advantageous affection; and if we find such qualities in the object, the affection will certainly arise. Thus indirectly the prospect of advantage may tend to raise any affection; but if these qualities be not found or apprehended in the object, no volition of ours, nor desire, will ever raise any affection in us.

But more particularly, that desire of the good of others, which we approve as virtuous, cannot be alleged to be voluntarily raised from prospect of any pleasure accompanying the affection itself: for it is plain that our benevolence is not always accompanied with pleasure; nay, it is often attended with pain, when the object is in distress. Desire in general is rather uneasy than pleasant. It is true, indeed, all the passions and affections justify themselves; while they continue, (as Malebranche expresses it) we generally approve our being thus affected on this occasion, as an innocent disposition, or a just one, and condemn a person who would be otherwise affected on the like occasion. So the sorrowful, the angry, the jealous, the compassionate, approve their several passions on the apprehended occasion; but we should not therefore conclude, that sorrow, anger, jealousy or pity are pleasant, or chosen for their concomitant pleasure. The case is plainly thus: the frame of our nature on the occasions which move these passions, determines us to be thus affected, and to approve our affection at least as innocent. Uneasiness generally attends our desires of any kind; and this sensation tends to fix our attention, and to continue the desire. But the desire does not terminate upon the removal of the pain accompanying the desire, but upon some other event: the concomitant pain is what we seldom reflect upon, unless when it is very violent. Nor does any desire or affection terminate upon the pleasure which may accompany the affection; much less is it raised by an act of our will, with a view to obtain this pleasure.

The same reflection will show, that we do not by an act of our will raise in ourselves that benevolence which we approve as virtuous, with a view to obtain future pleasures of self-approbation by our moral sense. Could we raise affections in this manner, we should be engaged to any affection by the prospect of an interest equivalent to this of self-approbation, such as wealth or sensual pleasure, which with many tempers are more powerful; and yet we universally own, that *that* disposition to do good offices to others, which is raised by these motives, is not virtuous: how can we then imagine, that the virtuous benevolence is brought upon us by a motive equally *selfish*?

*   *   *

v.   The other scheme is more plausible: that benevolence is not raised by any volition upon prospect of advantage; but that we desire the happiness of others, as conceiving it necessary to procure some pleasant sensations which we expect to feel upon seeing others happy; and that for like reason we have aversion to their misery. This connection between the happiness of others and our pleasure, say they, is chiefly felt among friends, parents and children, and eminently virtuous characters. But this benevolence flows as directly from self-love as any other desire.

To show that this scheme is not true in fact, let us consider, that if in our benevolence we only desired the happiness of others as the means of this pleasure to ourselves, whence is it that no man approves the desire of the happiness of others as a means of procuring wealth or sensual pleasure to ourselves? If a person had wagered concerning the future happiness of a man of such veracity, that he would sincerely confess whether he were happy or not; would this wagerer's desire of the happiness of another, in order to win the wager, be approved as virtuous? If not, wherein does this desire differ from the former? except that in one case there is one pleasant sensation expected, and in the other case other sensations: for by increasing or diminishing the sum wagered, the interest in this case may be made either greater or less than that in the other.

Reflecting on our own minds again will best discover the truth. Many have never thought upon this connection: nor do we ordinarily intend the obtaining of any such pleasure when we do generous offices. We all often feel delight upon seeing others happy, but during our pursuit of their happiness we have no intention of obtaining this delight. We often feel the pain of compassion; but were our sole ultimate intention or desire the freeing ourselves from this pain, would the Deity offer to us either wholly to blot out all memory of the person in distress, to take away this connection, so that we should be easy during the misery of our friend on the one hand, or on the other would relieve him from his misery, we should be as ready to choose the former way as the latter; since either of them would free us from our pain, which upon this scheme is the sole end proposed by the compassionate person. – Don't we find in ourselves that our desire does not terminate upon the removal of our own pain?

Were this our sole intention, we would run away, shut our eyes, or divert our thoughts from the miserable object, as the readiest way of removing our pain: this we seldom do, nay, we crowd about such objects, and voluntarily expose ourselves to this pain, unless calm reflection upon our inability to relieve the miserable, countermand our inclination, or some selfish affection, as fear of danger, overpower it.

To make this yet clearer, suppose that the Deity should declare to a good man that he should be suddenly annihilated, but at the instant of his exit it should be left to his choice whether his friend, his children, or his country should be made happy or miserable for the future, when he himself could have no sense of either pleasure or pain from their state. Pray would he be any more indifferent about their state now, that he neither hoped or feared any thing to himself from it, than he was in any prior period of his life? Nay, is it not a pretty common opinion among us, that after our decease we know nothing of what befalls those who survive us? How comes it then that we do not lose, at the approach of death, all concern for our families, friends, or country? Can there be any instance given of our desiring any thing only as the means of private good, as violently when we know that we shall not enjoy this good many minutes, as if we expected the possession of this good for many years? Is this the way we compute the value of annuities?

How the disinterested desire of the good of others should seem inconceivable, it is hard to account: perhaps it is owing to the attempts of some great men to give definitions of simple ideas. – *Desire*, say they, is uneasiness, or uneasy sensation upon the absence of any good. – Whereas desire is as distinct from uneasiness, as volition is from sensation. Don't they themselves often speak of our desiring to remove uneasiness? Desire then is different from uneasiness, however a sense of uneasiness accompanies it, as extension does the idea of colour, which yet is a very distinct idea. Now wherein lies the impossibility of desiring the happiness of another without conceiving it as the means of obtaining any thing farther, even as we desire our own happiness without farther view? If any allege, that we desire our own happiness as the means of removing the uneasiness we feel in the absence of happiness, then at least the desire of removing our own uneasiness is an ultimate desire: and why may we not have other ultimate desires?

'But can any being be concerned about the absence of an event which gives it no uneasiness?' Perhaps superior natures desire without uneasy sensation. But what if we cannot? We may be uneasy while a desired event is in suspense, and yet not desire this event only as the means of removing this uneasiness: nay, if we did not desire the event without view to this uneasiness, we should never have brought the uneasiness upon ourselves by desiring it. So likewise we may feel delight upon the existence of a desired event, when yet we did not desire the event only as the means of obtaining this delight; even as we often receive delight from events which we had an aversion to.

Notes

1   Tragedy of Hamlet.
2   Cf. Hobbes, *Human Nature*, ch. IX.

3

From *Enquiry Concerning the Principles of Morals*

David Hume

Section I

134. There has been a controversy started of late, much better worth examination, concerning the general foundation of Morals; whether they be derived from Reason, or from Sentiment; whether we attain the knowledge of them by a chain of argument and induction, or by an immediate feeling and finer internal sense; whether, like all sound judgement of truth and falsehood, they should be the same to every rational intelligent being; or whether, like the perception of beauty and deformity, they be founded entirely on the particular fabric and constitution of the human species.

The ancient philosophers, though they often affirm, that virtue is nothing but conformity to reason, yet, in general, seem to consider morals as deriving their existence from taste and sentiment. On the other hand, our modern enquirers, though they also talk much of the beauty of virtue, and deformity of vice, yet have commonly endeavoured to account for these distinctions by metaphysical reasonings, and by deductions from the most abstract principles of the understanding. Such confusion reigned in these subjects, that an opposition of the greatest consequence could prevail between one system and another, and even in the parts of almost each individual system; and yet nobody, till very lately, was ever sensible of it. The elegant Lord Shaftesbury, who first gave occasion to remark this distinction, and who, in general, adhered to the principles of the ancients, is not, himself, entirely free from the same confusion.

David Hume, *Enquiries*, edited by L. A. Selby-Bigge; third edition editor, P. H. Nidditch (Oxford: Clarendon Press, 1975), pp. 170–5, 212–32, 250–78.

135. It must be acknowledged, that both sides of the question are susceptible of specious arguments. Moral distinctions, it may be said, are discernible by pure *reason*: else, whence the many disputes that reign in common life, as well as in philosophy, with regard to this subject: the long chain of proofs often produced on both sides; the examples cited, the authorities appealed to, the analogies employed, the fallacies detected, the inferences drawn, and the several conclusions adjusted to their proper principles. Truth is disputable; not taste: what exists in the nature of things is the standard of our judgement; what each man feels within himself is the standard of sentiment. Propositions in geometry may be proved, systems in physics may be controverted; but the harmony of verse, the tenderness of passion, the brilliancy of wit, must give immediate pleasure. No man reasons concerning another's beauty; but frequently concerning the justice or injustice of his actions. In every criminal trial the first object of the prisoner is to disprove the facts alleged, and deny the actions imputed to him: the second to prove, that, even if these actions were real, they might be justified, as innocent and lawful. It is confessedly by deductions of the understanding, that the first point is ascertained: how can we suppose that a different faculty of the mind is employed in fixing the other?

136. On the other hand, those who would resolve all moral determinations into *sentiment*, may endeavour to show, that it is impossible for reason ever to draw conclusions of this nature. To virtue, say they, it belongs to be *amiable*, and vice *odious*. This forms their very nature or essence. But can reason or argumentation distribute these different epithets to any subjects, and pronounce beforehand, that this must produce love, and that hatred? Or what other reason can we ever assign for these affections, but the original fabric and formation of the human mind, which is naturally adapted to receive them?

The end of all moral speculations is to teach us our duty; and, by proper representations of the deformity of vice and beauty of virtue, beget correspondent habits, and engage us to avoid the one, and embrace the other. But is this ever to be expected from inferences and conclusions of the understanding, which of themselves have no hold of the affections nor set in motion the active powers of men? They discover truths: but where the truths which they discover are indifferent, and beget no desire or aversion, they can have no influence on conduct and behaviour. What is honourable, what is fair, what is becoming, what is noble, what is generous, takes possession of the heart, and animates us to embrace and maintain it. What is intelligible, what is evident, what is probable, what is true, procures only the cool assent of the understanding; and gratifying a speculative curiosity, puts an end to our researches.

Extinguish all the warm feelings and prepossessions in favour of virtue, and all disgust or aversion to vice: render men totally indifferent towards these distinctions; and morality is no longer a practical study, nor has any tendency to regulate our lives and actions.

137. These arguments on each side (and many more might be produced) are so plausible, that I am apt to suspect, they may, the one as well as the other, be solid and satisfactory, and that *reason* and *sentiment* concur in almost all moral determinations and conclusions. The final sentence, it is probable, which pronounces characters and actions amiable or odious, praise-worthy or blameable; that which stamps on them the mark of honour or infamy, approbation or censure; that which renders morality an active principle and constitutes virtue our happiness, and vice our misery: it is probable, I say, that this final sentence depends on some internal sense or feeling, which nature has made universal in the whole species. For what else can have an influence of this nature? But in order to pave the way for such a sentiment, and give a proper discernment of its object, it is often necessary, we find, that much reasoning should precede, that nice distinctions be made, just conclusions drawn, distant comparisons formed, complicated relations examined, and general facts fixed and ascertained. Some species of beauty, especially the natural kinds, on their first appearance, command our affection and approbation; and where they fail of this effect, it is impossible for any reasoning to redress their influence, or adapt them better to our taste and sentiment. But in many orders of beauty, particularly those of the finer arts, it is requisite to employ much reasoning, in order to feel the proper sentiment; and a false relish may frequently be corrected by argument and reflection. There are just grounds to conclude, that moral beauty partakes much of this latter species, and demands the assistance of our intellectual faculties, in order to give it a suitable influence on the human mind.

138. But though this question, concerning the general principles of morals, be curious and important, it is needless for us, at present, to employ farther care in our researches concerning it. For if we can be so happy, in the course of this enquiry, as to discover the true origin of morals, it will then easily appear how far either sentiment or reason enters into all determinations of this nature. In order to attain this purpose, we shall endeavour to follow a very simple method: we shall analyse that complication of mental qualities, which form what, in common life, we call Personal Merit: we shall consider every attribute of the mind, which renders a man an object either of esteem and affection, or of hatred and contempt; every habit or sentiment or faculty, which, if ascribed to any person, implies either praise or blame, and may enter into any panegyric or satire of his character and manners. The quick sensibility, which, on this head, is so universal among mankind, gives a philosopher sufficient assurance, that he can never be considerably mistaken in framing the catalogue, or incur any danger of misplacing the objects of his contemplation: he needs only enter into his own breast for a moment, and consider whether or not he should desire to have this or that quality ascribed to him, and whether such or such an imputation would proceed from a friend or an enemy. The very nature of language guides us almost infallibly in forming a judgement of this nature; and as every tongue possesses one set of words which are taken in a good sense, and another in the opposite, the least acquaintance with the idiom suffices, without any reasoning, to direct us in collecting and arranging the estimable or blameable qualities of men. The only object of reasoning is to discover the circumstances on both sides, which are common to these qualities; to observe that particular in which the estimable qualities agree on the one hand, and the blameable on the other; and thence to reach the foundation of ethics, and find those universal principles, from which all censure or approbation is ultimately derived. As this is a question of fact, not of abstract science, we can only expect success, by following the experimental method, and deducing general maxims from a comparison of particular instances. The other scientific method, where a general abstract principle is first established, and is afterwards branched out into a variety of inferences and conclusions, may be more perfect in itself, but suits less the imperfection of human nature, and is a common source of illusion and mistake in this as well as in other subjects. Men are now cured of their passion for hypotheses and systems in natural philosophy, and will hearken to no arguments but those which are derived from experience. It is full time they should attempt a like reformation in all moral disquisitions; and reject every system of ethics, however subtle or ingenious, which is not founded on fact and observation.

We shall begin our enquiry on this head by the consideration of the social virtues, Benevolence and Justice. The explication of them will probably give us an opening by which the others may be accounted for.

Section V

Why utility pleases

Part I

172. It seems so natural a thought to ascribe to their utility the praise, which we bestow on the social virtues, that one would expect to meet with this principle everywhere in moral writers, as the chief foundation of their reasoning and enquiry. In common life, we may observe, that the circumstance of utility is always appealed to; nor is it supposed, that a greater eulogy can be given to any man, than to display his usefulness to the public, and enumerate the services, which he has performed to mankind and society. What praise, even of an inanimate form, if the regularity and elegance of its parts destroy not its fitness for any useful purpose! And how satisfactory an apology for any disproportion or seeming deformity, if we can show the necessity of that particular construction for the use intended! A ship appears more beautiful to an artist, or one moderately skilled in navigation, where its prow is wide and swelling beyond its poop, than if it were framed with a precise geometrical regularity, in contradiction to all the laws of mechanics. A building, whose doors and windows were exact squares, would hurt the eye by that very proportion; as ill adapted to the figure of a human creature, for whose service the fabric was intended. What wonder then, that a man, whose habits and conduct are hurtful to society, and dangerous or pernicious to every one who has an intercourse with him, should, on that account, be an object of disapprobation, and communicate to every spectator the strongest sentiment of disgust and hatred.[1]

But perhaps the difficulty of accounting for these effects of usefulness, or its contrary, has kept philosophers from admitting them into their systems of ethics, and has induced them rather to employ any other principle, in explaining the origin of moral good and evil. But it is no just reason for rejecting any principle, confirmed by experience, that we cannot give a satisfactory account of its origin, nor are able to resolve it into other more general principles. And if we would employ a little thought on the present subject, we need be at no loss to account for the influence of utility, and to deduce it from principles, the most known and avowed in human nature.

173. From the apparent usefulness of the social virtues, it has readily been inferred by sceptics, both ancient and modern, that all moral distinctions arise from education, and were, at first, invented, and afterwards encouraged, by the art of politicians, in order to render men tractable, and subdue their natural ferocity and selfishness, which incapacitated them for society. This principle, indeed, of precept and education, must so far be owned to have a powerful influence, that it may frequently increase or diminish, beyond their natural standard, the sentiments of approbation or dislike; and may even, in particular instances, create, without any natural principle, a new sentiment of this kind; as is evident in all superstitious practices and observances: But that *all* moral affection or dislike arises from this origin, will never surely be allowed by any judicious enquirer. Had nature made no such distinction, founded on the original constitution of the mind, the words, *honourable* and *shameful, lovely* and *odious, noble* and *despicable*, had never had place in any language; nor could politicians, had they invented these terms, ever have been able to render them intelligible, or make them convey any idea to the audience. So that nothing can be more superficial than this paradox of the sceptics; and it were well, if, in the abstruser studies of logic and metaphysics, we could as easily obviate the cavils of that sect, as in the practical and more intelligible sciences of politics and morals.

The social virtues must, therefore, be allowed to have a natural beauty and amiableness, which, at first, antecedent to all precept or education, recommends them to the esteem of uninstructed mankind, and engages their affections. And as the public utility of these virtues is the chief circumstance, whence they derive their merit, it follows, that the end, which they have a tendency to promote, must be some way agreeable to us, and take hold of some natural affection. It must please, either from considerations of self-interest, or from more generous motives and regards.

174.   It has often been asserted, that, as every man has a strong connexion with society, and perceives the impossibility of his solitary subsistence, he becomes, on that account, favourable to all those habits or principles, which promote order in society, and insure to him the quiet possession of so inestimable a blessing. As much as we value our own happiness and welfare, as much must we applaud the practice of justice and humanity, by which alone the social confederacy can be maintained, and every man reap the fruits of mutual protection and assistance.

This deduction of morals from self-love, or a regard to private interest, is an obvious thought, and has not arisen wholly from the wanton sallies and sportive assaults of the sceptics. To mention no others, Polybius, one of the gravest and most judicious, as well as most moral writers of antiquity, has assigned this selfish origin to all our sentiments of virtue.[2] But though the solid practical sense of that author, and his aversion to all vain subtilties, render his authority on the present subject very considerable; yet is not this an affair to be decided by authority, and the voice of nature and experience seems plainly to oppose the selfish theory.

175. We frequently bestow praise on virtuous actions, performed in very distant ages and remote countries; where the utmost subtilty of imagination would not discover any appearance of self-interest, or find any connexion of our present happiness and security with events so widely separated from us.

A generous, a brave, a noble deed, performed by an adversary, commands our approbation; while in its consequences it may be acknowledged prejudicial to our particular interest.

Where private advantage concurs with general affection for virtue, we readily perceive and avow the mixture of these distinct sentiments, which have a very different feeling and influence on the mind. We praise, perhaps, with more alacrity, where the generous humane action contributes to our particular interest: But the topics of praise, which we insist on, are very wide of this circumstance. And we may attempt to bring over others to our sentiments, without endeavouring to convince them, that they reap any advantage from the actions which we recommend to their approbation and applause.

Frame the model of a praiseworthy character, consisting of all the most amiable moral virtues: Give instances, in which these display themselves after an eminent and extraordinary manner: You readily engage the esteem and approbation of all your audience, who never so much as enquire in what age and country the person lived, who possessed these noble qualities: A circumstance, however, of all others, the most material to self-love, or a concern for our own individual happiness.

Once on a time, a statesman, in the shock and contest of parties, prevailed so far as to procure, by his eloquence, the banishment of an able adversary; whom he secretly followed, offering him money for his support during his exile, and soothing him with topics of consolation in his misfortunes. *Alas!* cries the banished statesman, *with what regret must I leave my friends in this city, where even enemies are so generous!* Virtue, though in an enemy, here pleased him: And we also give it the just tribute of praise and approbation; nor do we retract these sentiments, when we hear, that the action passed at Athens, about two thousand years ago, and that the persons' names were Eschines and Demosthenes.

What is that to me? There are few occasions, when this question is not pertinent: And had it that universal, infallible influence supposed, it would turn into ridicule every composition, and almost every conversation, which contain any praise or censure of men and manners.

176. It is but a weak subterfuge, when pressed by these facts and arguments, to say, that we transport ourselves, by the force of imagination, into distant ages and countries, and consider the advantage, which we should have reaped from these characters, had we been contemporaries, and had any commerce with the persons. It is not conceivable, how a *real* sentiment or passion can ever arise from a known *imaginary* interest; especially when our *real* interest is still kept in view, and is often acknowledged to be entirely distinct from the imaginary, and even sometimes opposite to it.

A man, brought to the brink of a precipice, cannot look down without trembling; and the sentiment of *imaginary* danger actuates him, in opposition to the opinion and belief of *real* safety. But the imagination is here assisted by the presence of a striking object; and yet prevails not, except it be also aided by novelty, and the unusual appearance of the object. Custom soon reconciles us to heights and precipices, and wears off these false and delusive terrors. The reverse is observable in the estimates which we form of characters and manners; and the more we habituate ourselves to an accurate scrutiny of morals, the more delicate feeling do we acquire of the most minute distinctions between vice and virtue. Such frequent occasion, indeed, have we, in common life, to pronounce all kinds of moral determinations, that no object of this kind can be new or unusual to us; nor could any *false* views or prepossessions maintain their ground against an experience, so common and familiar. Experience being chiefly what forms the associations of ideas, it is impossible that any association could establish and support itself, in direct opposition to that principle.

177. Usefulness is agreeable, and engages our approbation. This is a matter of fact, confirmed by daily observation. But, *useful?* For what? For somebody's interest, surely. Whose interest then? Not our own only: For our approbation frequently extends farther. It must, therefore, be the interest of those, who are served by the character or action approved of; and these we may conclude, however remote, are not totally indifferent to us. By opening up this principle, we shall discover one great source of moral distinctions.

Part II
178. Self-love is a principle in human nature of such extensive energy, and the interest of each individual is, in general, so closely connected with that of the community, that those philosophers were excusable, who fancied that all our concern for the public might be resolved into a concern for our own happiness and preservation. They saw every moment,

instances of approbation or blame, satisfaction or displeasure towards characters and actions; they denominated the objects of these sentiments, *virtues*, or *vices*; they observed, that the former had a tendency to increase the happiness, and the latter the misery of mankind; they asked, whether it were possible that we could have any general concern for society, or any disinterested resentment of the welfare or injury of others; they found it simpler to consider all these sentiments as modifications of self-love; and they discovered a pretence, at least, for this unity of principle, in that close union of interest, which is so observable between the public and each individual.

But notwithstanding this frequent confusion of interests, it is easy to attain what natural philosophers, after Lord Bacon, have affected to call the *experimentum crucis*, or that experiment which points out the right way in any doubt or ambiguity. We have found instances, in which private interest was separate from public; in which it was even contrary: And yet we observed the moral sentiment to continue, notwithstanding this disjunction of interests. And wherever these distinct interests sensibly concurred, we always found a sensible increase of the sentiment, and a more warm affection to virtue, and detestation of vice, or what we properly call, *gratitude* and *revenge*. Compelled by these instances, we must renounce the theory, which accounts for every moral sentiment by the principle of self-love. We must adopt a more public affection, and allow, that the interests of society are not, even on their own account, entirely indifferent to us. Usefulness is only a tendency to a certain end; and it is a contradiction in terms, that anything pleases as means to an end, where the end itself no wise affects us. If usefulness, therefore, be a source of moral sentiment, and if this usefulness be not always considered with a reference to self; it follows, that everything, which contributes to the happiness of society, recommends itself directly to our approbation and good-will. Here is a principle, which accounts, in great part, for the origin of morality: And what need we seek for abstruse and remote systems, when there occurs one so obvious and natural?[3]

179.   Have we any difficulty to comprehend the force of humanity and benevolence? Or to conceive, that the very aspect of happiness, joy, prosperity, gives pleasure; that of pain, suffering, sorrow, communicates uneasiness? The human countenance, says Horace,[4] borrows smiles or tears from the human countenance. Reduce a person to solitude, and he loses all enjoyment, except either of the sensual or speculative kind; and that because the movements of his heart are not forwarded by correspondent movements in his fellow-creatures. The signs of sorrow

and mourning, though arbitrary, affect us with melancholy; but the natural symptoms, tears and cries and groans, never fail to infuse compassion and uneasiness. And if the effects of misery touch us in so lively a manner; can we be supposed altogether insensible or indifferent towards its causes; when a malicious or treacherous character and behaviour are presented to us?

We enter, I shall suppose, into a convenient, warm, well-contrived apartment: We necessarily receive a pleasure from its very survey; because it presents us with the pleasing ideas of ease, satisfaction, and enjoyment. The hospitable, good-humoured, humane landlord appears. This circumstance surely must embellish the whole; nor can we easily forbear reflecting, with pleasure, on the satisfaction which results to every one from his intercourse and good-offices.

His whole family, by the freedom, ease, confidence, and calm enjoyment, diffused over their countenances, sufficiently express their happiness. I have a pleasing sympathy in the prospect of so much joy, and can never consider the source of it, without the most agreeable emotions.

He tells me, that an oppressive and powerful neighbour had attempted to dispossess him of his inheritance, and had long disturbed all his innocent and social pleasures. I feel an immediate indignation arise in me against such violence and injury.

But it is no wonder, he adds, that a private wrong should proceed from a man, who had enslaved provinces, depopulated cities, and made the field and scaffold stream with human blood. I am struck with horror at the prospect of so much misery, and am actuated by the strongest antipathy against its author.

180.   In general, it is certain, that, wherever we go, whatever we reflect on or converse about, everything still presents us with the view of human happiness or misery, and excites in our breast a sympathetic movement of pleasure or uneasiness. In our serious occupations, in our careless amusements, this principle still exerts its active energy.

A man who enters the theatre, is immediately struck with the view of so great a multitude, participating of one common amusement; and experiences, from their very aspect, a superior sensibility or disposition of being affected with every sentiment, which he shares with his fellow-creatures.

He observes the actors to be animated by the appearance of a full audience, and raised to a degree of enthusiasm, which they cannot command in any solitary or calm moment.

Every movement of the theatre, by a skilful poet, is communicated, as it were by magic, to the spectators; who weep, tremble, resent, rejoice, and are inflamed with all the variety of passions, which actuate the several personages of the drama.

Where any event crosses our wishes, and interrupts the happiness of the favourite characters, we feel a sensible anxiety and concern. But where their sufferings proceed from the treachery, cruelty, or tyranny of an enemy, our breasts are affected with the liveliest resentment against the author of these calamities.

It is here esteemed contrary to the rules of art to represent anything cool and indifferent. A distant friend, or a confident, who has no immediate interest in the catastrophe, ought, if possible, to be avoided by the poet; as communicating a like indifference to the audience, and checking the progress of the passions.

Few species of poetry are more entertaining than *pastoral*; and every one is sensible, that the chief source of its pleasure arises from those images of a gentle and tender tranquillity, which it represents in its personages, and of which it communicates a like sentiment to the reader. Sannazarius, who transferred the scene to the sea-shore, though he presented the most magnificent object in nature, is confessed to have erred in his choice. The idea of toil, labour, and danger, suffered by the fishermen, is painful; by an unavoidable sympathy, which attends every conception of human happiness or misery.

When I was twenty, says a French poet, Ovid was my favourite: Now I am forty, I declare for Horace. We enter, to be sure, more readily into sentiments, which resemble those we feel every day: But no passion, when well represented, can be entirely indifferent to us; because there is none, of which every man has not, within him, at least the seeds and first principles. It is the business of poetry to bring every affection near to us by lively imagery and representation, and make it look like truth and reality: A certain proof, that, wherever that reality is found, our minds are disposed to be strongly affected by it.

181.   Any recent event or piece of news, by which the fate of states, provinces, or many individuals is affected, is extremely interesting even to those whose welfare is not immediately engaged. Such intelligence is propagated with celerity, heard with avidity, and enquired into with attention and concern. The interest of society appears, on this occasion, to be in some degree the interest of each individual. The imagination is sure to be affected; though the passions excited may not always be so strong and steady as to have great influence on the conduct and behaviour.

The perusal of a history seems a calm entertainment; but would be no entertainment at all, did not our hearts beat with correspondent movements to those which are described by the historian.

Thucydides and Guicciardin support with difficulty our attention; while the former describes the trivial rencounters of the small cities of Greece, and the latter the harmless wars of Pisa. The few persons interested and the small interest fill not the imagination, and engage not the affections. The deep distress of the numerous Athenian army before Syracuse; the danger which so nearly threatens Venice; these excite compassion; these move terror and anxiety.

The indifferent, uninteresting style of Suetonius, equally with the masterly pencil of Tacitus, may convince us of the cruel depravity of Nero or Tiberius: But what a difference of sentiment! While the former coldly relates the facts; and the latter sets before our eyes the venerable figures of a Soranus and a Thrasea, intrepid in their fate, and only moved by the melting sorrows of their friends and kindred. What sympathy then touches every human heart! What indignation against the tyrant, whose causeless fear or unprovoked malice gave rise to such detestable barbarity!

182.   If we bring these subjects nearer: If we remove all suspicion of fiction and deceit: What powerful concern is excited, and how much superior, in many instances, to the narrow attachments of self-love and private interest! Popular sedition, party zeal, a devoted obedience to factious leaders; these are some of the most visible, though less laudable effects of this social sympathy in human nature.

The frivolousness of the subject too, we may observe, is not able to detach us entirely from what carries an image of human sentiment and affection.

When a person stutters, and pronounces with difficulty, we even sympathize with this trivial uneasiness, and suffer for him. And it is a rule in criticism, that every combination of syllables or letters, which gives pain to the organs of speech in the recital, appears also from a species of sympathy harsh and disagreeable to the ear. Nay, when we run over a book with our eye, we are sensible of such unharmonious composition; because we still imagine, that a person recites it to us, and suffers from the pronunciation of these jarring sounds. So delicate is our sympathy!

Easy and unconstrained postures and motions are always beautiful: An air of health and vigour is agreeable: Clothes which warm, without burthening the body; which cover, without imprisoning the limbs, are well-fashioned. In every judgement of beauty, the feelings of the person affected enter into consideration, and communicate to the spectator similar touches of pain or pleasure.[5] What wonder, then, if we can pronounce no judgement concerning the character and conduct of men, without considering the tendencies of their actions, and the happiness or misery which thence arises to society? What association of ideas would ever operate, were that principle here totally unactive.[6]

183.   If any man from a cold insensibility, or narrow selfishness of temper, is unaffected with the images of human happiness or misery, he must be equally indifferent to the images of vice and virtue: As, on the other hand, it is always found, that a warm concern for the interests of our species is attended with a delicate feeling of all moral distinctions; a strong resentment of injury done to men; a lively approbation of their welfare. In this particular, though great superiority is observable of one man above another; yet none are so entirely indifferent to the interest of their fellow-creatures, as to perceive no distinctions of moral good and evil, in consequence of the different tendencies of actions and principles. How, indeed, can we suppose it possible in any one, who wears a human heart, that if there be subjected to his censure, one character or system of conduct, which is beneficial, and another which is pernicious, to his species or community, he will not so much as give a cool preference to the former, or ascribe to it the smallest merit or regard? Let us suppose such a person ever so selfish; let private interest have ingrossed ever so much his attention; yet in instances, where that is not concerned, he must unavoidably feel *some* propensity to the good of mankind, and make it an object of choice, if everything else be equal. Would any man, who is walking along, tread as willingly on another's gouty toes, whom he has no quarrel with, as on the hard flint and pavement? There is here surely a difference in the case. We surely take into consideration the happiness and misery of others, in weighing the several motives of action, and incline to the former, where no private regards draw us to seek our own promotion or advantage by the injury of our fellow-creatures. And if the principles of humanity are capable, in many instances, of influencing our actions, they must, at all times, have *some* authority over our sentiments, and give us a general approbation of what is useful to society, and blame of what is dangerous or pernicious. The degrees of these sentiments may be the subject of controversy; but the reality of their existence, one should think, must be admitted in every theory or system.

184.   A creature, absolutely malicious and spiteful, were there any such in nature, must be worse than indifferent to the images of vice and virtue. All his sentiments must be inverted, and directly opposite to those, which prevail in the human species. Whatever contributes to the good of mankind, as it crosses the constant bent of his wishes and desires, must produce uneasiness and disapprobation; and on the contrary, whatever is the source of disorder and misery in society, must, for the same reason, be regarded with pleasure and complacency. Timon, who probably from his affected spleen more than any inveterate malice, was denominated the manhater, embraced Alcibiades with great fondness. *Go on my boy!* cried he, *acquire the confidence of the people: You will one day, I foresee, be the cause of great calamities to them.*[7] Could we admit the two principles of the Manicheans, it is an infallible consequence, that their sentiments of human actions, as well as of everything else, must be totally opposite, and that every instance of justice and humanity, from its necessary tendency, must please the one deity and displease the other. All mankind so far resemble the good principle, that, where interest or revenge or envy perverts not our disposition, we are always inclined, from our natural philanthropy, to give the preference to the happiness of society, and consequently to virtue above its opposite. Absolute, unprovoked, disinterested malice has never perhaps place in any human breast; or if it had, must there pervert all the sentiments of morals, as well as the feelings of humanity. If the cruelty of Nero be allowed entirely voluntary, and not rather the effect of constant fear and resentment; it is evident that Tigellinus, preferably to Seneca or Burrhus, must have possessed his steady and uniform approbation.

185.   A statesman or patriot, who serves our own country in our own time, has always a more passionate regard paid to him, than one whose beneficial influence operated on distant ages or remote nations; where the good, resulting from his generous humanity, being less connected with us, seems more obscure, and affects us with a less lively sympathy. We may own the merit to be equally great, though our sentiments are not raised to an equal height, in both cases. The judgement here corrects the inequalities of our internal emotions and perceptions; in like manner, as it preserves us from error, in the several variations of images, presented to our external senses. The same object, at a double distance, really throws on the eye a picture of but half the bulk; yet we imagine that it appears of the same size in both situations; because we know that on our approach to it, its image would expand on the eye, and that the difference consists not in the object itself, but in our position with regard to it. And, indeed, without such a correction of appearances, both in internal and external sentiment, men could never think or talk steadily on any subject; while their fluctuating situations produce a continual variation on objects, and throw them into such different and contrary lights and positions.[8]

186.   The more we converse with mankind, and the greater social intercourse we maintain, the more shall we be familiarized to these general preferences and distinctions, without which our conversation and discourse could scarcely be rendered intelligible to each other. Every man's interest is peculiar to himself, and the aversions and desires, which result from it, cannot be supposed to affect others in a like degree. General language, therefore, being formed for general use, must be moulded on some more general views, and must affix the epithets of praise or blame, in conformity to sentiments, which arise from the general interests of the community. And if these sentiments, in most men, be not so strong as those, which have a reference to private good; yet still they must make some distinction, even in persons the most depraved and selfish; and must attach the notion of good to a beneficent conduct, and of evil to the contrary. Sympathy, we shall allow, is much fainter than our concern for ourselves, and sympathy with persons remote from us much fainter than that with persons near and contiguous; but for this very reason it is necessary for us, in our calm judgements and discourse concerning the characters of men, to neglect all these differences, and render our sentiments more public and social. Besides, that we ourselves often change our situation in this particular, we every day meet with persons who are in a situation different from us, and who could never converse with us were we to remain constantly in that position and point of view, which is peculiar to ourselves. The intercourse of sentiments, therefore, in society and conversation, makes us form some general unalterable standard, by which we may approve or disapprove of characters and manners. And though the heart takes not part entirely with those general notions, nor regulates all its love and hatred, by the universal abstract differences of vice and virtue, without regard to self, or the persons with whom we are more intimately connected; yet have these moral differences a considerable influence, and being sufficient, at least, for discourse, serve all our purposes in company, in the pulpit, on the theatre, and in the schools.[9]

187. Thus, in whatever light we take this subject, the merit, ascribed to the social virtues, appears still uniform, and arises chiefly from that regard, which the natural sentiment of benevolence engages us to pay to the interests of mankind and society. If we consider the principles of the human make, such as they appear to daily experience and observation, we must, *a priori*, conclude it impossible for such a creature as man to be totally indifferent to the well or ill-being of his fellow-creatures, and not readily, of himself, to pronounce, where nothing gives him any particular bias, that what promotes their happiness is good, what tends to their misery is evil, without any farther regard or consideration. Here then are the faint rudiments, at least, or outlines, of a *general* distinction between actions; and in proportion as the humanity of the person is supposed to encrease, his connexion with those who are injured or benefited, and his lively conception of their misery or happiness; his consequent censure or approbation acquires proportionable vigour. There is no necessity, that a generous action, barely mentioned in an old history or remote gazette, should communicate any strong feelings of applause and admiration. Virtue, placed at such a distance, is like a fixed star, which, though to the eye of reason it may appear as luminous as the sun in his meridian, is so infinitely removed as to affect the senses, neither with light nor heat. Bring this virtue nearer, by our acquaintance or connexion with the persons, or even by an eloquent recital of the case; our hearts are immediately caught, our sympathy enlivened, and our cool approbation converted into the warmest sentiments of friendship and regard. These seem necessary and infallible consequences of the general principles of human nature, as discovered in common life and practice.

188.   Again; reverse these views and reasonings: Consider the matter *a posteriori*; and weighing the consequences, enquire if the merit of social virtue be not, in a great measure, derived from the feelings of humanity, with which it affects the spectators. It appears to be matter of fact, that the circumstance of *utility*, in all subjects, is a source of praise and approbation: That it is constantly appealed to in all moral decisions concerning the merit and demerit of actions: That it is the *sole* source of that high regard paid to justice, fidelity, honour, allegiance, and chastity: That it is inseparable from all the other social virtues, humanity, generosity, charity, affability, lenity, mercy, and moderation: And, in a word, that it is a foundation of the chief part of morals, which has a reference to mankind and our fellow-creatures.

189.   It appears also, that, in our general approbation of characters and manners, the useful tendency of the social virtues moves us not by any regards to self-interest, but has an influence much more universal and extensive. It appears that a tendency to public good, and to the promoting of peace, harmony, and order in society, does always, by affecting the benevolent principles of our frame, engage us on the side of the social virtues. And it appears, as an additional confirmation, that these principles of humanity and sympathy enter so deeply into all our sentiments, and have so powerful an influence, as may enable them to excite the strongest censure and applause. The present theory is the simple result of all these inferences, each of which seems founded on uniform experience and observation.

190.   Were it doubtful, whether there were any such principle in our nature as humanity or a concern for others, yet when we see, in numberless instances, that whatever has a tendency to promote the interests of society, is so highly approved of, we ought thence to learn the force of the benevolent principle; since it is impossible for anything to please as means to an end, where the end is totally indifferent. On the other hand, were it doubtful, whether there were, implanted in our nature, any general principle of moral blame and approbation, yet when we see, in numberless instances, the influence of humanity, we ought thence to conclude, that it is impossible, but that everything which promotes the interest of society must communicate pleasure, and what is pernicious give uneasiness. But when these different reflections and observations concur in establishing the same conclusion, must they not bestow an undisputed evidence upon it?

It is however hoped, that the progress of this argument will bring a farther confirmation of the present theory, by showing the rise of other sentiments of esteem and regard from the same or like principles.

Notes

1   We ought not to imagine, because an inanimate object may be useful as well as a man, that therefore it ought also, according to this system, to merit the appellation of *virtuous*. The sentiments, excited by utility, are, in the two cases, very different; and the one is mixed with affection, esteem, approbation, &c., and not the other. In like manner, an inanimate object may have good colour and proportions as well as a human figure. But can we ever be in love with the former? There are a numerous set of passions and sentiments, of which thinking rational beings are, by the original constitution of nature, the only proper objects: and though the very same qualities be transferred to an insensible, inanimate being, they will not excite the same sentiments. The beneficial qualities of herbs and minerals are, indeed, sometimes called their *virtues*; but this is an effect of the caprice of language, which ought not to be regarded in reasoning. For though there be a species of approbation attending even inanimate objects, when beneficial, yet this sentiment is so weak, and so different from that which is directed to beneficent magistrates or statesmen; that they ought not to be ranked under the same class or appellation.

A very small variation of the object, even where the same qualities are preserved, will destroy a sentiment. Thus, the same beauty, transferred to a different sex, excites no amorous passion, where nature is not extremely perverted.

2   Undutifulness to parents is disapproved of by mankind, προορωμένους τὸ μέλλον, καὶ συλλογιξομένους ὅτι τὸ παραπλήσιον ἑκάστοις αὐτῶν συγκυρήσει. Ingratitude for a like reason (though he seems there to mix a more generous regard) συναγανακτοῦνταζ μὲν τῷ πέλαζ, ἀναφέρονταζ δ᾽ ἐπ᾽ αὐτοὺζ τὸ παραπλήσιον, ἐξ ὧν ὑπογίγνεταί τιζ ἔννοια παρ᾽ ἑκάστῳ τῆζ τοῦ καθήκοντοζ δυνάμεωζ καὶ θεωρίαζ. Lib. vi. cap. 4 (ed. Gronovius). Perhaps the historian only meant, that our sympathy and humanity was more

enlivened, by our considering the similarity of our case with that of the person suffering; which is a just sentiment.

3   It is needless to push our researches so far as to ask, why we have humanity or a fellow-feeling with others. It is sufficient, that this is experienced to be a principle in human nature. We must stop somewhere in our examination of causes; and there are, in every science, some general principles, beyond which we cannot hope to find any principle more general. No man is absolutely indifferent to the happiness and misery of others. The first has a natural tendency to give pleasure; the second, pain. This every one may find in himself. It is not probable, that these principles can be resolved into principles more simple and universal, whatever attempts may have been made to that purpose. But if it were possible, it belongs not to the present subject; and we may here safely consider these principles as original: happy, if we can render all the consequences sufficiently plain and perspicuous!

4   'Uti ridentibus arrident, ita flentibus adflent
                 Humani vultus.' – Hor.

5   'Decentior equus cujus astricta sunt ilia; sed idem velocior. Pulcher aspectu sit athleta, cujus lacertos exercitatio expressit; idem certamini paratior. Nunquam enim *species* ab *utilitate* dividitur. Sed hoc quidem discernere modici judicii est.' – Quintilian, *Inst*. lib. viii. cap. 3.

6   In proportion to the station which a man possesses, according to the relations in which he is placed; we always expect from him a greater or less degree of good, and when disappointed, blame his inutility; and much more do we blame him, if any ill or prejudice arise from his conduct and behaviour. When the interests of one country interfere with those of another, we estimate the merits of a statesman by the good or ill, which results to his own country from his measures and councils, without regard to the prejudice which he brings on its enemies and rivals. His fellow-citizens are the objects, which lie nearest the eye, while we determine his character. And as nature has implanted in every one a superior affection to his own country, we never expect any regard to distant nations, where a competition arises. Not to mention, that, while every man consults the good of his own community, we are sensible, that the general interest of mankind is better promoted, than by any loose indeterminate views to the good of a species, whence no beneficial action could ever result, for want of.a duly limited object, on which they could exert themselves.

7   Plutarch *in vita Alc*.

8   For a like reason, the tendencies of actions and characters, not their real accidental consequences, are alone regarded in our moral determinations or general judgements; though in our real feeling or sentiment, we cannot help paying greater regard to one whose station, joined to virtue, renders him really useful to society, than to one, who exerts the social virtues only in good intentions and benevolent affections. Separating the character from the fortune, by an easy and necessary effort of thought, we pronounce these persons alike, and give them the same general praise. The judgement corrects or endeavours to correct the appearance: But is not able entirely to prevail over sentiment.

Why is this peach-tree said to be better than that other; but because it produces more or better fruit? And would not the same praise be given it, though snails or vermin had destroyed the peaches, before they came to full maturity? In morals too, is not *the tree known by the fruit?* And cannot we easily distinguish between nature and accident, in the one case as well as in the other?

9   It is wisely ordained by nature, that private connexions should commonly prevail over universal views and considerations; otherwise our affections and actions would be dissipated and lost, for want of a proper limited object. Thus a small benefit done to ourselves, or our near friends, excites more lively sentiments of love and approbation than a great benefit done to a distant commonwealth: But still we know here, as in all the senses, to correct these inequalities by reflection, and retain a general standard of vice and virtue, founded chiefly on general usefulness.

Section VII

Of qualities immediately agreeable to ourselves

203.   Whoever has passed an evening with serious melancholy people, and has observed how suddenly the conversation was animated, and what sprightliness diffused itself over the countenance, discourse, and behaviour of every one, on the accession of a good-humoured, lively companion; such a one will easily allow that cheerfulness carries great merit with it, and naturally conciliates the good-will of mankind. No quality, indeed, more readily communicates itself to all around; because no one has a greater propensity to display itself, in jovial talk and pleasant entertainment. The flame spreads through the whole circle; and the most sullen and morose are often caught by it. That the melancholy hate the merry, even though Horace says it, I have some difficulty to allow; because I have always observed that, where the jollity is moderate and decent, serious people are so much the more delighted, as it dissipates the gloom with which they are commonly oppressed, and gives them an unusual enjoyment.

From this influence of cheerfulness, both to communicate itself and to engage approbation, we may perceive that there is another set of mental qualities, which, without any utility or any tendency to farther good, either of the community or of the possessor, diffuse a satisfaction on the beholders, and procure friendship and regard. Their immediate sensation, to the person possessed of them, is agreeable. Others enter into the same humour, and catch the sentiment, by a contagion or natural sympathy; and as we cannot forbear loving whatever pleases, a kindly emotion arises towards the person who communicates so much satisfaction. He is a more animating spectacle; his presence diffuses over us more serene complacency and enjoyment; our imagination, entering into his feelings and disposition, is affected in a more agreeable manner than if a melancholy, dejected, sullen, anxious temper were presented to us. Hence the affection and approbation which attend the former: the aversion and disgust, with which we regard the latter.[1]

Few men would envy the character which Caesar gives of Cassius:

> He loves no play,
> As thou do'st, Anthony: he hears no music:
> Seldom he smiles; and smiles in such a sort,
> As if he mock'd himself, and scorn'd his spirit
> That could be mov'd to smile at any thing.

Not only such men, as Caesar adds, are commonly *dangerous*, but also, having little enjoyment within themselves, they can never become agreeable to others, or contribute to social entertainment. In all polite nations and ages, a relish for pleasure, if accompanied with temperance and decency, is esteemed a considerable merit, even in the greatest men; and becomes still more requisite in those of inferior rank and character. It is an agreeable representation, which a French writer gives of the situation of his own mind in this particular, *Virtue I love*, says he, *without austerity: Pleasure without effeminacy: And life, without fearing its end.*[2]

204.   Who is not struck with any signal instance of greatness of mind or dignity of character; with elevation of sentiment, disdain of slavery, and with that noble pride and spirit, which arises from conscious virtue? The sublime, says Longinus, is often nothing but the echo or image of magnanimity; and where this quality appears in any one, even though a syllable be not uttered, it excites our applause and admiration; as may be observed of the famous silence of Ajax in the Odyssey, which expresses more noble disdain and resolute indignation than any language can convey.[3]

Were I Alexander, said Parmenio, *I would accept of these offers made by* Darius. *So would I too*, replied Alexander, *were I* Parmenio. This saying is admirable, says Longinus, from a like principle.[4]

Go! cries the same hero to his soldiers, when they refused to follow him to the Indies, *go tell your countrymen, that you left* Alexander *completing the conquest of the world*. 'Alexander,' said the Prince of Condé, who always admired this passage, 'abandoned by his soldiers, among barbarians, not yet fully subdued, felt in himself such a dignity and right of empire, that he could not believe it possible that any one would refuse to obey him.

Whether in Europe or in Asia, among Greeks or Persians, all was indifferent to him: wherever he found men, he fancied he should find subjects.'

The confident of Medea in the tragedy recommends caution and submission; and enumerating all the distresses of that unfortunate heroine, asks her, what she has to support her against her numerous and implacable enemies. *Myself,* replies she; *Myself I say, and it is enough.* Boileau justly recommends this passage as an instance of true sublime.[5]

When Phocion, the modest, the gentle Phocion, was led to execution, he turned to one of his fellow-sufferers, who was lamenting his own hard fate, *Is it not glory enough for you,* says he, *that you die with* Phocion?[6]

Place in opposition the picture which Tacitus draws of Vitellius, fallen from empire, prolonging his ignominy from a wretched love of life, delivered over to the merciless rabble; tossed, buffeted, and kicked about; constrained, by their holding a poinard under his chin, to raise his head, and expose himself to every contumely. What abject infamy! What low humiliation! Yet even here, says the historian, he discovered some symptoms of a mind not wholly degenerate. To a tribune, who insulted him, he replied, *I am still your emperor.*[7]

We never excuse the absolute want of spirit and dignity of character, or a proper sense of what is due to one's self, in society and the common intercourse of life. This vice constitutes what we properly call *meanness;* when a man can submit to the basest slavery, in order to gain his ends; fawn upon those who abuse him; and degrade himself by intimacies and familiarities with undeserving inferiors. A certain degree of generous pride or self-value is so requisite, that the absence of it in the mind displeases, after the same manner as the want of a nose, eye, or any of the most material feature of the face or member of the body.[8]

205. The utility of courage, both to the public and to the person possessed of it, is an obvious foundation of merit. But to any one who duly considers of the matter, it will appear that this quality has a peculiar lustre, which it derives wholly from itself, and from that noble elevation inseparable from it. Its figure, drawn by painters and by poets, displays, in each feature, a sublimity and daring confidence; which catches the eye, engages the affections, and diffuses, by sympathy, a like sublimity of sentiment over every spectator.

Under what shining colours does Demosthenes[9] represent Philip; where the orator apologizes for his own administration, and justifies that pertinacious love of liberty, with which he had inspired the Athenians. 'I beheld Philip,' says he, 'he with whom was your contest, resolutely, while in pursuit of empire and dominion, exposing himself to every wound; his eye gored, his neck wrested, his arm, his thigh pierced, whatever part of his body fortune should seize on, that cheerfully relinquishing; provided that, with what remained, he might live in honour and renown. And shall it be said that he, born in Pella, a place heretofore mean and ignoble, should be inspired with so high an ambition and thirst of fame: while you, Athenians, &c.' These praises excite the most lively admiration; but the views presented by the orator, carry us not, we see, beyond the hero himself, nor ever regard the future advantageous consequences of his valour.

The martial temper of the Romans, inflamed by continual wars, had raised their esteem of courage so high, that, in their language, it was called *virtue*, by way of excellence and of distinction from all other moral qualities. *The* Suevi, in the opinion of Tacitus,[10] *dressed their hair with a laudable intent: not for the purpose of loving or being loved; they adorned themselves only for their enemies, and in order to appear more terrible.* A sentiment of the historian, which would sound a little oddly in other nations and other ages.

The Scythians, according to Herodotus,[11] after scalping their enemies, dressed the skin like leather, and used it as a towel; and whoever had the most of those towels was most esteemed among them. So much had martial bravery, in that nation, as well as in many others, destroyed the sentiments of humanity; a virtue surely much more useful and engaging.

It is indeed observable, that, among all uncultivated nations, who have not as yet had full experience of the advantages attending beneficence, justice, and the social virtues, courage is the predominant excellence; what is most celebrated by poets, recommended by parents and instructors, and admired by the public in general. The ethics of Homer are, in this particular, very different from those of Fénelon, his elegant imitator; and such as were well suited to an age, when one hero, as remarked by Thucydides,[12] could ask another, without offence, whether he were a robber or not. Such also very lately was the system of ethics which prevailed in many barbarous parts of Ireland; if we may credit Spenser, in his judicious account of the state of that kingdom.[13]

206.   Of the same class of virtues with courage is that undisturbed philosophical tranquillity, superior to pain, sorrow, anxiety, and each assault of adverse fortune. Conscious of his own virtue, say the philosophers, the sage elevates himself above every accident of life; and securely placed in the temple of wisdom, looks down on inferior mortals engaged in pursuit of honours, riches, reputation, and every frivolous enjoyment. These pretensions, no doubt, when stretched to the utmost, are by far too magnificent for human nature. They carry, however, a grandeur with them, which seizes the spectator, and strikes him with admiration. And the nearer we can approach in practice to this sublime tranquillity and indifference (for we must distinguish it from a stupid insensibility), the more secure enjoyment shall we attain within ourselves, and the more greatness of mind shall we discover to the world. The philosophical tranquillity may, indeed, be considered only as a branch of magnanimity.

Who admires not Socrates; his perpetual serenity and contentment, amidst the greatest poverty and domestic vexations; his resolute contempt of riches, and his magnanimous care of preserving liberty, while he refused all assistance from his friends and disciples, and avoided even the dependence of an obligation? Epictetus had not so much as a door to his little house or hovel; and therefore, soon lost his iron lamp, the only furniture which he had worth taking. But resolving to disappoint all robbers for the future, he supplied its place with an earthen lamp, of which he very peaceably kept possession ever after.

Among the ancients, the heroes in philosophy, as well as those in war and patriotism, have a grandeur and force of sentiment, which astonishes our narrow souls, and is rashly rejected as extravagant and supernatural. They, in their turn, I allow, would have had equal reason to consider as romantic and incredible, the degree of humanity, clemency, order, tranquillity, and other social virtues, to which, in the administration of government, we have attained in modern times, had any one been then able to have made a fair representation of them. Such is the compensation, which nature, or rather education, has made in the distribution of excellencies and virtues, in those different ages.

207. The merit of benevolence, arising from its utility, and its tendency to promote the good of mankind, has been already explained, and is, no doubt, the source of a *considerable* part of that esteem, which is so universally paid to it. But it will also be allowed, that the very softness and tenderness of the sentiment, its engaging endearments, its fond expressions, its delicate attentions, and all that flow of mutual confidence and regard, which enters into a warm attachment of love and friendship: it will be allowed, I say, that these feelings, being delightful in themselves, are necessarily communicated to the spectators, and melt them into the same fondness and delicacy. The tear naturally starts in our eye on the apprehension of a warm sentiment of this nature: our breast heaves, our heart is agitated, and every humane tender principle of our frame is set in motion, and gives us the purest and most satisfactory enjoyment.

When poets form descriptions of Elysian fields, where the blessed inhabitants stand in no need of each other's assistance, they yet represent them as maintaining a constant intercourse of love and friendship, and sooth our fancy with the pleasing image of these soft and gentle passions. The idea of tender tranquillity in a pastoral Arcadia is agreeable from a like principle, as has been observed above.[14]

Who would live amidst perpetual wrangling, and scolding, and mutual reproaches? The roughness and harshness of these emotions disturb and displease us: we suffer by contagion and sympathy; nor can we remain indifferent spectators, even though certain that no pernicious consequences would ever follow from such angry passions.

208.   As a certain proof that the whole merit of benevolence is not derived from its usefulness, we may observe, that in a kind way of blame, we say, a person is *too good*; when he exceeds his part in society, and carries his attention for others beyond the proper bounds. In like manner, we say a man is *too high-spirited, too intrepid, too indifferent about fortune*: reproaches, which really, at bottom, imply more esteem than many panegyrics. Being accustomed to rate the merit and demerit of characters chiefly by their useful or pernicious tendencies, we cannot forbear applying the epithet of blame, when we discover a sentiment, which rises to a degree, that is hurtful; but it may happen, at the same time, that its noble elevation, or its engaging tenderness so seizes the heart, as rather to increase our friendship and concern for the person.[15]

The amours and attachments of Harry the IVth of France, during the civil wars of the league, frequently hurt his interest and his cause; but all the young, at least, and amorous, who can sympathize with the tender passions, will allow that this very weakness (for they will readily call it such) chiefly endears that hero, and interests them in his fortunes.

The excessive bravery and resolute inflexibility of Charles the XIIth ruined his own country, and infested all his neighbours; but have such splendour and greatness in their appearance, as strikes us with admiration; and they might, in some degree, be even approved of, if they betrayed not sometimes too evident symptoms of madness and disorder.

209.   The Athenians pretended to the first invention of agriculture and of laws: and always valued themselves extremely on the benefit thereby procured to the whole race of mankind. They also boasted, and with reason, of their warlike enterprises; particularly against those innumerable fleets and armies of Persians, which invaded Greece during the reigns of Darius and Xerxes. But though there be no comparison in point of utility, between these peaceful and military honours; yet we find, that the orators, who have writ such elaborate panegyrics on that famous city, have chiefly triumphed in displaying the warlike achievements. Lysias, Thucydides, Plato, and Isocrates discover, all of them, the same partiality; which, though condemned by calm reason and reflection, appears so natural in the mind of man.

It is observable, that the great charm of poetry consists in lively pictures of the sublime passions, magnanimity, courage, disdain of fortune; or those of the tender affections, love and friendship; which warm the heart, and diffuse over it similar sentiments and emotions. And though all kinds of passion, even the most disagreeable, such as grief and anger, are observed, when excited by poetry, to convey a satisfaction, from a mechanism of nature, not easy to be explained: Yet those more elevated or softer affections have a peculiar influence, and please from more than one cause or principle. Not to mention that they alone interest us in the fortune of the persons represented, or communicate any esteem and affection for their character.

And can it possibly be doubted, that this talent itself of poets, to move the passions, this pathetic and sublime of sentiment, is a very considerable merit; and being enhanced by its extreme rarity, may exalt the person possessed of it, above every character of the age in which he lives? The prudence, address, steadiness, and benign government of Augustus, adorned with all the splendour of his noble birth and imperial crown, render him but an unequal competitor for fame with Virgil, who lays nothing into the opposite scale but the divine beauties of his poetical genius.

The very sensibility to these beauties, or a delicacy of taste, is itself a beauty in any character; as conveying the purest, the most durable, and most innocent of all enjoyments.

210.   These are some instances of the several species of merit, that are valued for the immediate pleasure which they communicate to the person possessed of them. No views of utility or of future beneficial consequences enter into this sentiment of approbation; yet is it of a kind similar to that other sentiment, which arises from views of a public or private utility. The same social sympathy, we may observe, or fellow-feeling with human happiness or misery, gives rise to both; and this analogy, in all the parts of the present theory, may justly be regarded as a confirmation of it.

Notes

1   There is no man, who, on particular occasions, is not affected with all the disagreeable passions, fear, anger, dejection, grief, melancholy, anxiety, &c.

But these, so far as they are natural, and universal, make no difference between one man and another, and can never be the object of blame. It is only when the disposition gives a *propensity* to any of these disagreeable passions, that they disfigure the character, and by giving uneasiness, convey the sentiment of disapprobation to the spectator.

2   'J'aime la vertu, sans rudesse;
          J'aime le plaisir, sans molesse;
          J'aime la vie, et n'en crains point la fin.' – *St. Evremond.*

3   Cap. 9.

4   Idem.

5   Réflexion 10 sur Longin.

6   Plutarch in Phoc.

7   Tacit. hist. lib. iii. The author entering upon the narration, says, *Laniata veste, foedum spectaculum ducebatur, multis increpantibus, nullo inlacrimante:* deformitas exitus misericordiam abstulerat. To enter thoroughly into this method of thinking, we must make allowance for the ancient maxims, that no one ought to prolong his life after it became dishonourable; but, as he had always a right to dispose of it, it then became a duty to part with it.

8   The absence of virtue may often be a vice; and that of the highest kind; as in the instance of ingratitude, as well as meanness. Where we expect a beauty, the disappointment gives an uneasy sensation, and produces a real deformity. An abjectness of character, likewise, is disgustful and contemptible in another view. Where a man has no sense of value in himself, we are not likely to have any higher esteem of him. And if the same person, who crouches to his superiors, is insolent to his inferiors (as often happens), this contrariety of behaviour, instead of correcting the former vice, aggravates it extremely by the addition of a vice still more odious. See Section VIII.

9   Pro Corona.

10 De moribus Germ.

11 Lib. iv.

12 Lib. i.

13 It is a common use, says he, amongst their gentlemen's sons, that, as soon as they are able to use their weapons, they strait gather to themselves three or four stragglers or kern, with whom wandering a while up and down idly the country, taking only meat, he at last falleth into some bad occasion, that shall be offered; which being once made known, he is thenceforth counted a man of worth, in whom there is courage.

14 Sect. v. Part 2.

15 Cheerfulness could scarce admit of blame from its excess, were it not that dissolute mirth, without a proper cause or subject, is a sure symptom and characteristic of folly, and on that account disgustful.

Section VIII

Of qualities immediately agreeable to others[1]

211.   As the mutual shocks, in *society*, and the oppositions of interest and self-love have constrained mankind to establish the laws of *justice*, in order to preserve the advantages of mutual assistance and protection: in like manner, the eternal contrarieties, in *company*, of men's pride and self-conceit, have introduced the rules of Good Manners or Politeness, in order to facilitate the intercourse of minds, and an undisturbed commerce and conversation. Among well-bred people, a mutual deference is affected; contempt of others disguised; authority concealed; attention given to each in his turn; and an easy stream of conversation maintained, without vehemence, without interruption, without eagerness for victory, and without any airs of superiority. These attentions and regards are immediately *agreeable* to others, abstracted from any consideration of utility or beneficial tendencies: they conciliate affection, promote esteem, and extremely enhance the merit of the person who regulates his behaviour by them.

Many of the forms of breeding are arbitrary and casual; but the thing expressed by them is still the same. A Spaniard goes out of his own house before his guest, to signify that he leaves him master of all. In other countries, the landlord walks out last, as a common mark of deference and regard.

212.   But, in order to render a man perfect *good company*, he must have Wit and Ingenuity as well as good manners. What wit is, it may not be easy to define; but it is easy surely to determine that it is a quality immediately *agreeable* to others, and communicating, on its first appearance, a lively joy and satisfaction to every one who has any comprehension of it. The most profound metaphysics, indeed, might be employed in explaining the various kinds and species of wit; and many classes of it, which are now received on the sole testimony of taste and sentiment, might, perhaps, be resolved into more general principles. But this is sufficient for our present purpose, that it does affect taste and sentiment, and bestowing an immediate enjoyment, is a sure source of approbation and affection.

In countries where men pass most of their time in conversation, and visits, and assemblies, these *companionable* qualities, so to speak, are of high estimation, and form a chief part of personal merit. In countries where men live a more domestic life, and either are employed in business, or amuse themselves in a narrower circle of acquaintance, the more solid qualities are chiefly regarded. Thus, I have often observed, that, among the French, the first questions with regard to a stranger are, *Is he polite? Has he wit?* In our own country, the chief praise bestowed is always that of a *good-natured, sensible fellow.*

In conversation, the lively spirit of dialogue is *agreeable,* even to those who desire not to have any share in the discourse: hence the teller of long stories, or the pompous declaimer, is very little approved of. But most men desire likewise their turn in the conversation, and regard, with a very evil eye, that *loquacity* which deprives them of a right they are naturally so jealous of.

There is a sort of harmless *liars,* frequently to be met with in company, who deal much in the marvellous. Their usual intention is to please and entertain; but as men are most delighted with what they conceive to be truth, these people mistake extremely the means of pleasing, and incur universal blame. Some indulgence, however, to lying or fiction is given in *humorous* stories; because it is there really agreeable and entertaining, and truth is not of any importance.

Eloquence, genius of all kinds, even good sense, and sound reasoning, when it rises to an eminent degree, and is employed upon subjects of any considerable dignity and nice discernment; all these endowments seem immediately agreeable, and have a merit distinct from their usefulness. Rarity, likewise, which so much enhances the price of every thing, must set an additional value on these noble talents of the human mind.

213.   Modesty may be understood in different senses, even abstracted from chastity, which has been already treated of. It sometimes means that tenderness and nicety of honour, that apprehension of blame, that dread of intrusion or injury towards others, that Pudor, which is the proper guardian of every kind of virtue, and a sure preservative against vice and corruption. But its most usual meaning is when it is opposed to *impudence* and *arrogance,* and expresses a diffidence of our own judgement, and a due attention and regard for others. In young men chiefly, this quality is a sure sign of good sense; and is also the certain means of augmenting that endowment, by preserving their ears open to instruction, and making them still grasp after new attainments. But it has a further charm to every spectator; by flattering every man's vanity, and presenting the appearance of a docile pupil, who receives, with proper attention and respect, every word they utter.

Men have, in general, a much greater propensity to overvalue than undervalue themselves; notwithstanding the opinion of Aristotle.[2] This makes us more jealous of the excess on the former side, and causes us to regard, with a peculiar indulgence, all tendency to modesty and self-diffidence; as esteeming the danger less of falling into any vicious extreme of that nature. It is thus in countries where men's bodies are apt to exceed in corpulency, personal beauty is placed in a much greater degree of slenderness, than in countries where that is the most usual defect. Being so often struck with instances of one species of deformity, men think they can never keep at too great a distance from it, and wish always to have a leaning to the opposite side. In like manner, were the door opened to self-praise, and were Montaigne's maxim observed, that one should say as frankly, *I have sense, I have learning, I have courage, beauty, or wit*, as it is sure we often think so; were this the case, I say, every one is sensible that such a flood of impertinence would break in upon us, as would render society wholly intolerable. For this reason custom has established it as a rule, in common societies, that men should not indulge themselves in self-praise, or even speak much of themselves; and it is only among intimate friends or people of very manly behaviour, that one is allowed to do himself justice. Nobody finds fault with Maurice, Prince of Orange, for his reply to one who asked him, whom he esteemed the first general of the age, *The marquis of Spinola*, said he, *is the second*. Though it is observable, that the self-praise implied is here better implied, than if it had been directly expressed, without any cover or disguise.

He must be a very superficial thinker, who imagines that all instances of mutual deference are to be understood in earnest, and that a man would be more esteemable for being ignorant of his own merits and accomplishments. A small bias towards modesty, even in the internal sentiment, is favourably regarded, especially in young people; and a strong bias is required in the outward behaviour; but this excludes not a noble pride and spirit, which may openly display itself in its full extent, when one lies under calumny or oppression of any kind. The generous contumacy of Socrates, as Cicero calls it, has been highly celebrated in all ages; and when joined to the usual modesty of his behaviour, forms a shining character. Iphicrates, the Athenian, being accused of betraying the interests of his country, asked his accuser, *Would you*, says he, *have, on a like occasion, been guilty of that crime? By no means*, replied the other. *And can you then imagine*, cried the hero, *that* Iphicrates *would be guilty?*[3] In short, a generous spirit and self-value, well founded, decently disguised, and courageously supported under distress and calumny, is a great excellency, and seems to derive its merit from the noble elevation of its sentiment, or its immediate agreeableness to its possessor. In ordinary characters, we approve of a bias towards modesty, which is a quality immediately agreeable to others: the vicious excess of the former virtue, namely, insolence or haughtiness, is immediately disagreeable to others;

the excess of the latter is so to the possessor. Thus are the boundaries of these duties adjusted.

214. A desire of fame, reputation, or a character with others, is so far from being blameable, that it seems inseparable from virtue, genius, capacity, and a generous or noble disposition. An attention even to trivial matters, in order to please, is also expected and demanded by society; and no one is surprised, if he find a man in company to observe a greater elegance of dress and more pleasant flow of conversation, than when he passes his time at home, and with his own family. Wherein, then, consists Vanity, which is so justly regarded as a fault or imperfection? It seems to consist chiefly in such an intemperate display of our advantages, honours, and accomplishments; in such an importunate and open demand of praise and admiration, as is offensive to others, and encroaches too far on *their* secret vanity and ambition. It is besides a sure symptom of the want of true dignity and elevation of mind, which is so great an ornament in any character. For why that impatient desire of applause; as if you were not justly entitled to it, and might not reasonably expect that it would for ever attend you? Why so anxious to inform us of the great company which you have kept; the obliging things which were said to you; the honours, the distinctions which you met with; as if these were not things of course, and what we could readily, of ourselves, have imagined, without being told of them?

215.   Decency, or a proper regard to age, sex, character, and station in the world, may be ranked among the qualities which are immediately agreeable to others, and which, by that means, acquire praise and approbation. An effeminate behaviour in a man, a rough manner in a woman; these are ugly because unsuitable to each character, and different from the qualities which we expect in the sexes. It is as if a tragedy abounded in comic beauties, or a comedy in tragic. The disproportions hurt the eye, and convey a disagreeable sentiment to the spectators, the source of blame and disapprobation. This is that *indecorum*, which is explained so much at large by Cicero in his Offices.

Among the other virtues, we may also give Cleanliness a place; since it naturally renders us agreeable to others, and is no inconsiderable source of love and affection. No one will deny, that a negligence in this particular is a fault; and as faults are nothing but smaller vices, and this fault can have no other origin than the uneasy sensation which it excites in others; we may, in this instance, seemingly so trivial, clearly discover the origin of moral distinctions, about which the learned have involved themselves in such mazes of perplexity and error.

216.   But besides all the *agreeable* qualities, the origin of whose beauty we can, in some degree, explain and account for, there still remains something mysterious and inexplicable, which conveys an immediate satisfaction to the spectator, but how, or why, or for what reason, he cannot pretend to determine. There is a manner, a grace, an ease, a genteelness, an I-know-not-what, which some men possess above others, which is very different from external beauty and comeliness, and which, however, catches our affection almost as suddenly and powerfully. And though this *manner* be chiefly talked of in the passion between the sexes, where the concealed magic is easily explained, yet surely much of it prevails in all our estimation of characters, and forms no inconsiderable part of personal merit. This class of accomplishments, therefore, must be trusted entirely to the blind, but sure testimony of taste and sentiment; and must be considered as a part of ethics, left by nature to baffle all the pride of philosophy, and make her sensible of her narrow boundaries and slender acquisitions.

We approve of another, because of his wit, politeness, modesty, decency, or any agreeable quality which he possesses; although he be not of our acquaintance, nor has ever given us any entertainment, by means of these accomplishments. The idea, which we form of their effect on his ac-quaintance, has an agreeable influence on our imagination, and gives us the sentiment of approbation. This principle enters into all the judgements which we form concerning manners and characters.

Notes

1 It is the nature and, indeed, the definition of virtue, that it is *a quality of the mind agreeable to or approved of by every one who considers or contemplates it*. But some qualities produce pleasure, because they are useful to society, or useful or agreeable to the person himself; others produce it more immediately, which is the case with the class of virtues here considered.
2 Ethic. ad Nicomachum.
3 Quinctil. lib. v. cap. 12.

Section IX

Conclusion

Part I

217. It may justly appear surprising that any man in so late an age, should find it requisite to prove, by elaborate reasoning, that Personal Merit consists altogether in the possession of mental qualities, *useful* or *agreeable* to the *person himself* or to *others*. It might be expected that this principle would have occurred even to the first rude, unpractised enquirers concerning morals, and been received from its own evidence, without any argument or disputation. Whatever is valuable in any kind, so naturally classes itself under the division of *useful* or *agreeable*, the *utile* or the *dulce*, that it is not easy to imagine why we should ever seek further, or consider the question as a matter of nice research or inquiry. And as every thing useful or agreeable must possess these qualities with regard either to the *person himself* or to *others*, the complete delineation or description of merit seems to be performed as naturally as a shadow is cast by the sun, or an image is reflected upon water. If the ground, on which the shadow is cast, be not broken and uneven; nor the surface from which the image is reflected, disturbed and confused; a just figure is immediately presented, without any art or attention. And it seems a reasonable presumption, that systems and hypotheses have perverted our natural understanding, when a theory, so simple and obvious, could so long have escaped the most elaborate examination.

218.   But however the case may have fared with philosophy, in common life these principles are still implicitly maintained; nor is any other topic of praise or blame ever recurred to, when we employ any panegyric or satire, any applause or censure of human action and be-haviour. If we observe men, in every intercourse of business or pleasure, in every discourse and conversation, we shall find them nowhere, except in the schools, at any loss upon this subject. What so natural, for instance, as the following dialogue? You are very happy, we shall suppose one to say, addressing himself to another, that you have given your daughter to Cleanthes. He is a man of honour and humanity. Every one, who has any intercourse with him, is sure of *fair* and *kind* treatment.[1] I congratulate you too, says another, on the promising expectations of this son-in-law; whose assiduous application to the study of the laws, whose quick penetration and early knowledge both of men and business, prognosticate the greatest honours and advancement.[2] You surprise me, replies a third, when you talk of Cleanthes as a man of business and application. I met him lately in a circle of the gayest company, and he was the very life and soul of our conversation: so much wit with good manners; so much gallantry without affectation; so much ingenious knowledge so genteelly delivered, I have never before observed in any one.[3] You would admire him still more, says a fourth, if you knew him more familiarly. That cheerfulness, which you might remark in him, is not a sudden flash struck out by company: it runs through the whole tenor of his life, and preserves a perpetual serenity on his countenance, and tranquillity in his soul. He has met with severe trials, misfortunes as well as dangers; and by his greatness of mind, was still superior to all of them.[4] The image, gentlemen, which you have here delineated of Cleanthes, cried I, is that of accomplished merit. Each of you has given a stroke of the pencil to his figure; and you have unawares exceeded all the pictures drawn by Gratian or Castiglione. A philosopher might select this character as a model of perfect virtue.

219.   And as every quality which is useful or agreeable to ourselves or others is, in common life, allowed to be a part of personal merit; so no other will ever be received, where men judge of things by their natural, unprejudiced reason, without the delusive glosses of superstition and false religion. Celibacy, fasting, penance, mortification, self-denial, humility, silence, solitude, and the whole train of monkish virtues; for what reason are they everywhere rejected by men of sense, but because they serve to no manner of purpose; neither advance a man's fortune in the world, nor render him a more valuable member of society; neither qualify him for the entertainment of company, nor increase his power of self-enjoyment? We observe, on the contrary, that they cross all these desirable ends; stupify the understanding and harden the heart, obscure the fancy and sour the temper. We justly, therefore, transfer them to the opposite column, and place them in the catalogue of vices; nor has any superstition force sufficient among men of the world, to pervert entirely these natural sentiments. A gloomy, hair-brained enthusiast, after this death, may have a place in the calendar; but will scarcely ever be admitted, when alive, into intimacy and society, except by those who are as delirious and dismal as himself.

220.   It seems a happiness in the present theory, that it enters not into that vulgar dispute concerning the *degrees* of benevolence or self-love, which prevail in human nature; a dispute which is never likely to have any issue, both because men, who have taken part, are not easily convinced, and because the phenomena, which can be produced on either side, are so dispersed, so uncertain, and subject to so many interpretations, that it is scarcely possible accurately to compare them, or draw from them any determinate inference or conclusion. It is sufficient for our present purpose, if it be allowed, what surely, without the greatest absurdity cannot be disputed, that there is some benevolence, however small, infused into our bosom; some spark of friendship for human kind; some particle of the dove kneaded into our frame, along with the elements of the wolf and serpent. Let these generous sentiments be supposed ever so weak; let them be insufficient to move even a hand or finger of our body, they must still direct the determinations of our mind, and where everything else is equal, produce a cool preference of what is useful and serviceable to mankind, above what is pernicious and dangerous. A *moral distinction*, therefore, immediately arises; a general sentiment of blame and approbation; a tendency, however faint, to the objects of the one, and a proportionable aversion to those of the other. Nor will those reasoners, who so earnestly maintain the predominant selfishness of human kind, be any wise scandalized at hearing of the weak sentiments of virtue implanted in our nature. On the contrary, they are found as ready to maintain the one tenet as the other; and their spirit of satire (for such it appears, rather than of corruption) naturally gives rise to both opinions; which have, indeed, a great and almost an indissoluble connexion together.

221. Avarice, ambition, vanity, and all passions vulgarly, though improperly, comprised under the denomination of *self-love*, are here excluded from our theory concerning the origin of morals, not because they are too weak, but because they have not a proper direction for that purpose. The notion of morals implies some sentiment common to all mankind, which recommends the same object to general approbation, and makes every man, or most men, agree in the same opinion or decision concerning it. It also implies some sentiment, so universal and comprehensive as to extend to all mankind, and render the actions and conduct, even of the persons the most remote, an object of applause or censure, according as they agree or disagree with that rule of right which is established. These two requisite circumstances belong alone to the sentiment of humanity here insisted on. The other passions produce in every breast, many strong sentiments of desire and aversion, affection and hatred; but these neither are felt so much in common, nor are so comprehensive, as to be the foundation of any general system and established theory of blame or approbation.

222. When a man denominates another his *enemy*, his *rival*, his *antagonist*, his *adversary*, he is understood to speak the language of self-love, and to express sentiments, peculiar to himself, and arising from his particular circumstances and situation. But when he bestows on any man the epithets of *vicious* or *odious* or *depraved*, he then speaks another language, and expresses sentiments, in which he expects all his audience are to concur with him. He must here, therefore, depart from his private and particular situation, and must choose a point of view, common to him with others; he must move some universal principle of the human frame, and touch a string to which all mankind have an accord and symphony. If he mean, therefore, to express that this man possesses qualities, whose tendency is pernicious to society, he has chosen this common point of view, and has touched the principle of humanity, in which every man, in some degree, concurs. While the human heart is compounded of the same elements as at present, it will never be wholly indifferent to public good, nor entirely unaffected with the tendency of characters and manners. And though this affection of humanity may not generally be esteemed so strong as vanity or ambition, yet, being common to all men, it can alone be the foundation of morals, or of any general system of blame or praise. One man's ambition is not another's ambition, nor will the same event or object satisfy both; but the humanity of one man is the humanity of every one, and the same object touches this passion in all human creatures.

223.   But the sentiments, which arise from humanity, are not only the same in all human creatures, and produce the same approbation or censure; but they also comprehend all human creatures; nor is there any one whose conduct or character is not, by their means, an object to every one of censure or approbation. On the contrary, those other passions, commonly denominated selfish, both produce different sentiments in each individual, according to his particular situation; and also contemplate the greater part of mankind with the utmost indifference and unconcern. Whoever has a high regard and esteem for me flatters my vanity; whoever expresses contempt mortifies and displeases me; but as my name is known but to a small part of mankind, there are few who come within the sphere of this passion, or excite, on its account, either my affection or disgust. But if you represent a tyrannical, insolent, or barbarous behaviour, in any country or in any age of the world, I soon carry my eye to the pernicious tendency of such a conduct, and feel the sentiment of repugnance and displeasure towards it. No character can be so remote as to be, in this light, wholly indifferent to me. What is beneficial to society or to the person himself must still be preferred. And every quality or action, of every human being, must, by this means, be ranked under some class or denomination, expressive of general censure or applause.

What more, therefore, can we ask to distinguish the sentiments, dependent on humanity, from those connected with any other passion, or to satisfy us, why the former are the origin of morals, not the latter? Whatever conduct gains my approbation, by touching my humanity, procures also the applause of all mankind, by affecting the same principle in them; but what serves my avarice or ambition pleases these passions in me alone, and affects not the avarice and ambition of the rest of mankind. There is no circumstance of conduct in any man, provided it have a beneficial tendency, that is not agreeable to my humanity, however remote the person; but every man, so far removed as neither to cross nor serve my avarice and ambition, is regarded as wholly indifferent by those passions. The distinction, therefore, between these species of sentiment being so great and evident, language must soon be moulded upon it, and must invent a peculiar set of terms, in order to express those universal sentiments of censure or approbation, which arise from humanity, or from views of general usefulness and its contrary. Virtue and Vice become then known; morals are recognized; certain general ideas are framed of human conduct and behaviour; such measures are expected from men in such situations. This action is determined to be conformable to our abstract rule; that other, contrary. And by such universal principles are the particular sentiments of self-love frequently controlled and limited.[5]

224.   From instances of popular tumults, seditions, factions, panics, and of all passions, which are shared with a multitude, we may learn the influence of society in exciting and supporting any emotion; while the most ungovernable disorders are raised, we find, by that means, from the slightest and most frivolous occasions. Solon was no very cruel, though, perhaps, an unjust legislator, who punished neuters in civil wars; and few, I believe, would, in such cases, incur the penalty, were their affection and discourse allowed sufficient to absolve them. No selfishness, and scarce any philosophy, have there force sufficient to support a total coolness and indifference; and he must be more or less than man, who kindles not in the common blaze. What wonder then, that moral sentiments are found of such influence in life; though springing from principles, which may appear, at first sight, somewhat small and delicate? But these principles, we must remark, are social and universal; they form, in a manner, the *party* of humankind against vice or disorder, its common enemy. And as the benevolent concern for others is diffused, in a greater or less degree, over all men, and is the same in all, it occurs more frequently in discourse, is cherished by society and conversation, and the blame and approbation, consequent on it, are thereby roused from that lethargy into which they are probably lulled, in solitary and uncultivated nature. Other passions, though perhaps originally stronger, yet being selfish and private, are often overpowered by its force, and yield the dominion of our breast to those social and public principles.

225.   Another spring of our constitution, that brings a great addition of force to moral sentiment, is the love of fame; which rules, with such uncontrolled authority, in all generous minds, and is often the grand object of all their designs and undertakings. By our continual and earnest pursuit of a character, a name, a reputation in the world, we bring our own deportment and conduct frequently in review, and consider how they appear in the eyes of those who approach and regard us. This constant habit of surveying ourselves, as it were, in reflection, keeps alive all the sentiments of right and wrong, and begets, in noble natures, a certain reverence for themselves as well as others, which is the surest guardian of every virtue. The animal conveniencies and pleasures sink gradually in their value; while every inward beauty and moral grace is studiously acquired, and the mind is accomplished in every perfection, which can adorn or embellish a rational creature.

Here is the most perfect morality with which we are acquainted: here is displayed the force of many sympathies. Our moral sentiment is itself a feeling chiefly of that nature, and our regard to a character with others seems to arise only from a care of preserving a character with ourselves; and in order to attain this end, we find it necessary to prop our tottering judgement on the correspondent approbation of mankind.

226. But, that we may accommodate matters, and remove if possible every difficulty, let us allow all these reasonings to be false. Let us allow that, when we resolve the pleasure, which arises from views of utility, into the sentiments of humanity and sympathy, we have embraced a wrong hypothesis. Let us confess it necessary to find some other explication of that applause, which is paid to objects, whether inanimate, animate, or rational, if they have a tendency to promote the welfare and advantage of mankind. However difficult it be to conceive that an object is approved of on account of its tendency to a certain end, while the end itself is totally indifferent: let us swallow this absurdity, and consider what are the consequences. The preceding delineation or definition of Personal Merit must still retain its evidence and authority: it must still be allowed that every quality of the mind, which is *useful* or *agreeable* to the *person himself* or to *others*, communicates a pleasure to the spectator, engages his esteem, and is admitted under the honourable denomination of virtue or merit. Are not justice, fidelity, honour, veracity, allegiance, chastity, esteemed solely on account of their tendency to promote the good of society? Is not that tendency inseparable from humanity, benevolence, lenity, generosity, gratitude, moderation, tenderness, friendship, and all the other social virtues? Can it possibly be doubted that industry, discretion, frugality, secrecy, order, perseverance, forethought, judgement, and this whole class of virtues and accomplishments, of which many pages would not contain the catalogue; can it be doubted, I say, that the tendency of these qualities to promote the interest and happiness of their possessor, is the sole foundation of their merit? Who can dispute that a mind, which supports a perpetual serenity and cheerfulness, a noble dignity and undaunted spirit, a tender affection and good-will to all around; as it has more enjoyment within itself, is also a more animating and rejoicing spectacle, than if dejected with melancholy, tormented with anxiety, irritated with

rage, or sunk into the most abject baseness and degeneracy? And as to the qualities, immediately *agreeable to others*, they speak sufficiently for themselves; and he must be unhappy, indeed, either in his own temper, or in his situation and company, who has never perceived the charms of a facetious wit or flowing affability, of a delicate modesty or decent genteelness of address and manner.

227. I am sensible, that nothing can be more unphilosophical than to be positive or dogmatical on any subject; and that, even if *excessive* scepticism could be maintained, it would not be more destructive to all just reasoning and inquiry. I am convinced that, where men are the most sure and arrogant, they are commonly the most mistaken, and have there given reins to passion, without that proper deliberation and suspense, which can alone secure them from the grossest absurdities. Yet, I must confess, that this enumeration puts the matter in so strong a light, that I cannot, *at present*, be more assured of any truth, which I learn from reasoning and argument, than that personal merit consists entirely in the usefulness or agreeableness of qualities to the person himself possessed of them, or to others, who have any intercourse with him. But when I reflect that, though the bulk and figure of the earth have been measured and delineated, though the motions of the tides have been accounted for, the order and economy of the heavenly bodies subjected to their proper laws, and Infinite itself reduced to calculation; yet men still dispute concerning the foundation of their moral duties. When I reflect on this, I say, I fall back into diffidence and scepticism, and suspect that an hypothesis, so obvious, had it been a true one, would, long ere now, have been received by the unanimous suffrage and consent of mankind.

Notes

1   Qualities useful to others.
2   Qualities useful to the person himself.
3   Qualities immediately agreeable to others.
4   Qualities immediately agreeable to the person himself.
5   It seems certain, both from reason and experience, that a rude, untaught savage regulates chiefly his love and hatred by the ideas of private utility and injury, and has but faint conceptions of a general rule or system of behaviour. The man who stands opposite to him in battle, he hates heartily, not only for the present moment, which is almost unavoidable, but for ever after; nor is he satisfied without the most extreme punishment and vengeance. But we, accustomed to society, and to more enlarged reflections, consider, that this man is serving his own country and community; that any man, in the same

situation, would do the same; that we ourselves, in like circumstances, observe a like conduct; that, in general, human society is best supported on such maxims: and by these suppositions and views, we correct, in some measure, our ruder and narrower passions. And though much of our friendship and enmity be still regulated by private considerations of benefit and harm, we pay, at least, this homage to general rules, which we are accustomed to respect, that we commonly pervert our adversary's conduct, by imputing malice or injustice to him, in order to give vent to those passions, which arise from self-love and private interest. When the heart is full of rage, it never wants pretences of this nature; though sometimes as frivolous, as those from which Horace, being almost crushed by the fall of a tree, affects to accuse of parricide the first planter of it.

Part II

Contemporary Expressions

4

Virtues and Vices

Philippa Foot

I

For many years the subject of the virtues and vices was strangely neglected by moralists working within the school of analytic philosophy. The tacitly accepted opinion was that a study of the topic would form no part of the fundamental work of ethics; and since this opinion was apparently shared by philosophers such as Hume, Kant, Mill, G. E. Moore, W. D. Ross, and H. A. Prichard, from whom contemporary moral philosophy has mostly been derived, perhaps the neglect was not so surprising after all. However that may be, things have recently been changing. During the past ten or fifteen years several philosophers have turned their attention to the subject; notably G. H. von Wright and Peter Geach. Von Wright devoted a not at all perfunctory chapter to the virtues in his book *The Varieties of Goodness*[1] published in 1963, and Peter Geach's book called *The Virtues*[2] appeared in 1977. Meanwhile a number of interesting articles on the topic have come out in the journals.

In spite of this recent work, it is best when considering the virtues and vices to go back to Aristotle and Aquinas. I myself have found Plato less helpful, because the individual virtues and vices are not so clearly or consistently distinguished in his work. It is certain, in any case, that the most systematic account is found in Aristotle, and in the blending of Aristotelian and Christian philosophy found in St. Thomas. By and large Aquinas followed Aristotle – sometimes even heroically – where Aristotle gave an opinion, and where St. Thomas is on his own, as in developing

Philippa Foot, "Virtues and Vices," *Virtues and Vices and Other Essays in Moral Philosophy* (Berkeley, CA: University of California Press, 1978), pp. 1–18.

the doctrine of the theological virtues of faith, hope and charity, and in his theocentric doctrine of happiness, he still uses an Aristotelian framework where he can: as for instance in speaking of happiness as man's last end. However, there are different emphases and new elements in Aquinas's ethics: often he works things out in far more detail than Aristotle did, and it is possible to learn a great deal from Aquinas that one could not have got from Aristotle. It is my opinion that the *Summa Theologica* is one of the best sources we have for moral philosophy, and moreover that St. Thomas's ethical writings are as useful to the atheist as to the Catholic or other Christian believer.

There is, however, one minor obstacle to be overcome when one goes back to Aristotle and Aquinas for help in constructing a theory of virtues, namely a lack of coincidence between their terminology and our own. For when we talk about the virtues we are not taking as our subject everything to which Aristotle gave the name *aretē* or Aquinas *virtus*, and consequently not everything called a virtue in translations of these authors. 'The virtues' to us are the moral virtues whereas *aretē* and *virtus* refer also to arts, and even to excellences of the speculative intellect whose domain is theory rather than practice. And to make things more confusing we find some dispositions called moral virtues in translations from the Greek and Latin, although the class of virtues that Aristotle calls *aretai ēthikai* and Aquinas *virtutes morales* does not exactly correspond with our class of moral virtues. For us there are four cardinal moral virtues: courage, temperance, wisdom and justice. But Aristotle and Aquinas call only three of these virtues moral virtues; practical wisdom (Aristotle's *phronēsis* and Aquinas's *prudentia*) they class with the intellectual virtues, though they point out the close connexions between practical wisdom and what they call moral virtues; and sometimes they even use *aretē* and *virtus* very much as we use 'virtue'.

I will come back to Aristotle and Aquinas, and shall indeed refer to them frequently in this paper. But I want to start by making some remarks, admittedly fragmentary, about the concept of a moral virtue as we understand the idea.

First of all it seems clear that virtues are, in some general way, beneficial. Human beings do not get on well without them. Nobody can get on well if he lacks courage, and does not have some measure of temperance and wisdom, while communities where justice and charity are lacking are apt to be wretched places to live, as Russia was under the Stalinist terror, or Sicily under the Mafia. But now we must ask to whom the benefit goes, whether to the man who has the virtue or rather to those who have to do with him? In the case of some of the virtues the answer seems clear. Courage, temperance and wisdom benefit both the man who has these dispositions and other people as well; and moral failings such as pride, vanity, worldliness, and avarice harm both their possessor and others, though chiefly perhaps the former. But what about the virtues of charity and justice? These are directly concerned with the welfare of others, and with what is owed to them; and since each may require sacrifice of interest on the part of the virtuous man both may seem to be deleterious to their possessor and beneficial to others. Whether in fact it is so has, of course, been a matter of controversy since Plato's time or earlier. It is a reasonable opinion that on the whole a man is better off for being charitable and just, but this is not to say that circumstances may not arise in which he will have to sacrifice everything for charity or justice.

Nor is this the only problem about the relation between virtue and human good. For one very difficult question concerns the relation between justice and the common good. Justice, in the wide sense in which it is understood in discussions of the cardinal virtues, and in this paper, has to do with that to which someone has a right – that which he is owed in respect of non-interference and positive service – and rights may stand in the way of the pursuit of the common good. Or so at least it seems to those who reject utilitarian doctrines. This dispute cannot be settled here, but I shall treat justice as a virtue independent of charity, and standing as a possible limit on the scope of that virtue.

Let us say then, leaving unsolved problems behind us, that virtues are in general beneficial characteristics, and indeed ones that a human being needs to have, for his own sake and that of his fellows. This will not, however, take us far towards a definition of a virtue, since there are many other qualities of a man that may be similarly beneficial, as for instance bodily characteristics such as health and physical strength, and mental powers such as those of memory and concentration. What is it, we must ask, that differentiates virtues from such things?

As a first approximation to an answer we might say that while health and strength are excellences of the body, and memory and concentration of the mind, it is the will that is good in a man of virtue. But this suggestion is worth only as much as the explanation that follows it. What might we mean by saying that virtue belongs to the will?

In the first place we observe that it is primarily by his intentions that a man's moral dispositions are judged. If he does something unintentionally this is usually irrelevant to our estimate of his virtue. But of course this thesis must be qualified, because failures in performance rather than intention may show a lack of virtue. This will be so when, for instance, one man brings harm to another without realising he is doing it, but where his ignorance is itself culpable. Sometimes in such cases there will be a previous act or omission to which we can point as the source of the ignorance. Charity requires that we take care to find out how to render assistance where we are likely to be called on to do so, and thus, for example, it is contrary to charity to fail to find out about elementary first aid. But in an interesting class of cases in which it seems again to be performance rather than intention that counts in judging a man's virtue there is no possibility of shifting the judgement to previous intentions. For sometimes one man succeeds where another fails not because there is some specific difference in their previous conduct but rather because his heart lies in a different place; and the disposition of the heart is part of virtue.

Thus it seems right to attribute a kind of moral failing to some deeply discouraging and debilitating people who say, without lying, that they mean to be helpful; and on the other side to see virtue *par excellence* in one who is prompt and resourceful in doing good. In his novel *A Single Pebble* John Hersey describes such a man, speaking of a rescue in a swift flowing river:

> It was the head tracker's marvellous swift response that captured my admiration at first, his split second solicitousness when he heard a cry of pain, his finding in mid-air, as it were, the only way to save the injured boy. But there was more to it than that. His action, which could not have been mulled over in his mind, showed a deep, instinctive love of life, a compassion, an optimism, which made me feel very good . . .

What this suggests is that a man's virtue may be judged by his innermost desires as well as by his intentions; and this fits with our idea that a virtue such as generosity lies as much in someone's attitudes as in his actions. Pleasure in the good fortune of others is, one thinks, the sign of a generous spirit; and small reactions of pleasure and displeasure often the surest signs of a man's moral disposition.

None of this shows that it is wrong to think of virtues as belonging to the will; what it does show is that 'will' must here be understood in its widest sense, to cover what is wished for as well as what is sought.

A different set of considerations will, however, force us to give up any simple statement about the relation between virtue and will, and these considerations have to do with the virtue of wisdom. Practical wisdom, we said, was counted by Aristotle among the intellectual virtues, and while our *wisdom* is not quite the same as *phronēsis* or *prudentia* it too might seem to belong to the intellect rather than the will. Is not wisdom a matter of knowledge, and how can knowledge be a matter of intention or desire? The answer is that it isn't, so that there is good reason for thinking of wisdom as an intellectual virtue. But on the other hand wisdom has special connexions with the will, meeting it at more than one point.

In order to get this rather complex picture in focus we must pause for a little and ask what it is that we ourselves understand by wisdom: what the wise man knows and what he does. Wisdom, as I see it, has two parts. In the first place the wise man knows the means to certain good ends; and secondly he knows how much particular ends are worth. Wisdom in its first part is relatively easy to understand. It seems that there are some ends belonging to human life in general rather than to particular skills such as medicine or boatbuilding, ends having to do with such matters as friendship, marriage, the bringing up of children, or the choice of ways of life; and it seems that knowledge of how to act well in these matters belongs to some people but not to others. We call those who have this knowledge wise, while those who do not have it are seen as lacking wisdom. So, as both Aristotle and Aquinas insisted, wisdom is to be contrasted with cleverness because cleverness is the ability to take the right steps to any end, whereas wisdom is related only to good ends, and to human life in general rather than to the ends of particular arts.

Moreover, we should add, there belongs to wisdom only that part of knowledge which is within the reach of any ordinary adult human being: knowledge that can be acquired only by someone who is clever or who has access to special training is not counted as part of wisdom, and would not be so counted even if it could serve the ends that wisdom serves. It is therefore quite wrong to suggest that wisdom cannot be a moral virtue because virtue must be within the reach of anyone who really wants it and some people are too stupid to be anything but ignorant even about the most fundamental matters of human life. Some people are wise without being at all clever or well informed: they make good decisions and they know, as we say, 'what's what'.

In short wisdom, in what we called its first part, is connected with the will in the following ways. To begin with it presupposes good ends: the man who is wise does not merely know *how* to do good things such as looking after his children well, or strengthening someone in trouble, but must also want to do them. And then wisdom, in so far as it consists of knowledge which anyone can gain in the course of an ordinary life, is available to anyone who really wants it. As Aquinas put it, it belongs 'to a power under the direction of the will'.[3]

The second part of wisdom, which has to do with values, is much harder to describe, because here we meet ideas which are curiously elusive, such as the thought that some pursuits are more worthwhile than others, and some matters trivial and some important in human life. Since it makes good sense to say that most men waste a lot of their lives in ardent pursuit of what is trivial and unimportant it is not possible to explain the important and the trivial in terms of the amount of attention given to different subjects by the average man. But I have never seen, or been able to think out, a true account of this matter, and I believe that a complete account of wisdom, and of certain other virtues and vices must wait until this gap can be filled. What we can see is that one of the things a wise man knows and a foolish man does not is that such things as social position, and wealth, and the good opinion of the world, are too dearly bought at the cost of health or friendship or family ties. So we may say that a man who lacks wisdom 'has false values', and that vices such as vanity and worldliness and avarice are contrary to wisdom in a special way. There is always an element of false judgement about these vices, since the man who is vain for instance sees admiration as more important than it is, while the worldly man is apt to see the good life as one of wealth and power. Adapting Aristotle's distinction between the weak-willed man (the *akratēs*) who follows pleasure though he knows, in some sense, that he should not, and the licentious man (the *akolastos*) who sees the life of pleasure as the good life,[4] we may say that moral failings such as these are never purely 'akratic'. It is true that a man may criticise himself for his worldliness or vanity or love of money, but then it is his values that are the subject of his criticism.

Wisdom in this second part is, therefore, partly to be described in terms of apprehension, and even judgement, but since it has to do with a man's attachments it also characterises his will.

The idea that virtues belong to the will, and that this helps to distinguish them from such things as bodily strength or intellectual ability has, then, survived the consideration of the virtue of wisdom, albeit in a fairly complex and slightly attenuated form. And we shall find this idea useful again if we turn to another important distinction that must be made, namely that between virtues and other practical excellences such as arts and skills.

Aristotle has sometimes been accused, for instance by von Wright, of failing to see how different virtues are from arts or skills;[5] but in fact one finds, among the many things that Aristotle and Aquinas say about this difference, the observation that seems to go to the heart of the matter. In the matter of arts and skills, they say, voluntary error is preferable to involuntary error, while in the matter of virtues (what we call virtues) it is the reverse.[6] The last part of the thesis is actually rather hard to interpret, because it is not clear what is meant by the idea of involuntary viciousness. But we can leave this aside and still have all we need in order to distinguish arts or skills from virtues. If we think, for instance, of someone who deliberately makes a spelling mistake (perhaps when writing on the blackboard in order to explain this particular point) we see that this does not in any way count against his skill as a speller: 'I did it deliberately' rebuts an accusation of this kind. And what we can say without running into any difficulties is that there is no comparable rebuttal in the case of an accusation relating to lack of virtue. If a man acts unjustly or uncharitably, or in a cowardly or intemperate manner, 'I did it deliberately' cannot on any interpretation lead to exculpation. So, we may say, a virtue is not, like a skill or an art, a mere capacity: it must actually engage the will.

II

I shall now turn to another thesis about the virtues, which I might express by saying that they are *corrective*, each one standing at a point at which there is some temptation to be resisted or deficiency of motivation to be made good. As Aristotle put it, virtues are about what is difficult for men, and I want to see in what sense this is true, and then to consider a problem in Kant's moral philosophy in the light of what has been said.

Let us first think about courage and temperance. Aristotle and Aquinas contrasted these virtues with justice in the following respect. Justice was concerned with operation, and courage and temperance with passions.[7] What they meant by this seems to have been, primarily, that the man of courage does not fear immoderately nor the man of temperance have immoderate desires for pleasure, and that there was no corresponding moderation of a passion implied in the idea of justice. This particular account of courage and temperance might be disputed on the ground that a man's courage is measured by his action and not by anything as uncontrollable as fear; and similarly that the temperate man who must on occasion refuse pleasures need not *desire* them any less than the intemperate man. Be that as it may (and something will be said about it later) it is obviously true that courage and temperance have to do with particular springs of action as justice does not. Almost any desire can lead a man to act unjustly, not even excluding the desire to help a friend or to save a life, whereas a cowardly act must be motivated by fear or a desire for safety, and an act of intemperance by a desire for pleasure, perhaps even for a particular range of pleasures such as those of eating or drinking or sex. And now, going back to the idea of virtues as correctives, one may say that it is only because fear and the desire for pleasure often operate as temptations that courage and temperance exist as virtues at all. As things are we often want to run away not only where that is the right thing to do but also where we should stand firm; and we want pleasure not only where we should seek pleasure but also where we should not. If human nature had been different there would have been no need of a corrective disposition in either place, as fear and pleasure would have been good guides to conduct throughout life. So Aquinas says, about the passions

> They may incite us to something against reason, and so we need a curb, which we name *temperance*. Or they may make us shirk a course of action dictated by reason, through fear of dangers or hardships. Then a person needs to be steadfast and not run away from what is right; and for this *courage* is named.[8]

As with courage and temperance so with many other virtues: there is, for instance, a virtue of industriousness only because idleness is a temptation; and of humility only because men tend to think too well of themselves. Hope is a virtue because despair too is a temptation; it might have been that no one cried that all was lost except where he could really see it to be so, and in this case there would have been no virtue of hope.

With virtues such as justice and charity it is a little different, because they correspond not to any particular desire or tendency that has to be kept in check but rather to a deficiency of motivation; and it is this that they must make good. If people were as much attached to the good of others as they are to their own good there would no more be a general virtue of benevolence than there is a general virtue of self-love. And if people cared about the rights of others as they care about their own rights no virtue of justice would be needed to look after the matter, and rules about such things as contracts and promises would only need to be made public, like the rules of a game that everyone was eager to play.

On this view of the virtues and vices everything is seen to depend on what human nature is like, and the traditional catalogue of the two kinds of dispositions is not hard to understand. Nevertheless it may be defective, and anyone who accepts the thesis that I am putting forward will feel free to ask himself where the temptations and deficiencies that need correcting are really to be found. It is possible, for example, that the theory of human nature lying behind the traditional list of the virtues and vices puts too much emphasis on hedonistic and sensual impulses, and does not sufficiently take account of less straightforward inclinations such as the desire to be put upon and dissatisfied, or the unwillingness to accept good things as they come along.

It should now be clear why I said that virtues should be seen as correctives; and part of what is meant by saying that virtue is about things that are difficult for men should also have appeared. The further application of this idea is, however, controversial, and the following difficulty presents itself: that we both are and are not inclined to think that the harder a man finds it to act virtuously the more virtue he shows if he does act well. For on the one hand great virtue is needed where it is particularly hard to act virtuously; yet on the other it could be argued that difficulty in acting virtuously shows that the agent is imperfect in virtue: according to Aristotle, to take pleasure in virtuous action is the mark of true virtue, with the self-mastery of the one who finds virtue difficult only a second best. How then is this conflict to be decided? Who shows most courage, the one who wants to run away but does not, or the one who does not even want to run away? Who shows most charity, the one who finds it easy to make the good of others his object, or the one who finds it hard?

What is certain is that the thought that virtues are corrective does not constrain us to relate virtue to difficulty in each individual man. Since men in general find it hard to face great dangers or evils, and even small ones, we may count as courageous those few who without blindness or indifference are nevertheless fearless even in terrible circumstances. And when someone has a natural charity or generosity it is at least part of the virtue that he has; if natural virtue cannot be the whole of virtue this is because a kindly or fearless disposition could be disastrous without justice and wisdom, and because these virtues have to be learned, not because natural virtue is too easily acquired. I have argued that the virtues can be seen as correctives in relation to human nature in general but not that each virtue must present a difficulty to each and every man.

Nevertheless many people feel strongly inclined to say that it is for moral effort that moral praise is to be bestowed, and that in proportion as a man finds it easy to be virtuous so much the less is he to be morally admired for his good actions. The dilemma can be resolved only when we stop talking about difficulties standing in the way of virtuous action as if they were of only one kind. The fact is that some kinds of difficulties do indeed provide an occasion for much virtue, but that others rather show that virtue is incomplete.

To illustrate this point I shall first consider an example of honest action. We may suppose for instance that a man has an opportunity to steal, in circumstances where stealing is not morally permissible, but that he refrains. And now let us ask our old question. For one man it is hard to refrain from stealing and for another man it is not: which shows the greater virtue in acting as he should? It is not difficult to see in this case that it makes all the difference whether the difficulty comes from circumstances, as that a man is poor, or that his theft is unlikely to be detected, or whether it comes from something that belongs to his own character. The fact that a man is *tempted* to steal is something about him that shows a certain lack of honesty: of the thoroughly honest man we say that it 'never entered his head', meaning that it was never a real possibility for him. But the fact that he is poor is something that makes the occasion more *tempting*, and difficulties of this kind make honest action all the more virtuous.

A similar distinction can be made between different obstacles standing in the way of charitable action. Some circumstances, as that great sacrifice is needed, or that the one to be helped is a rival, give an occasion on which a man's charity is severely tested. Yet in given circumstances of this kind it is the man who acts easily rather than the one who finds it hard who shows the most charity. Charity is a virtue of attachment, and that sympathy for others which makes it easier to help them is part of the virtue itself.

These are fairly simple cases, but I am not supposing that it is always easy to say where the relevant distinction is to be drawn. What, for instance, should we say about the emotion of fear as an obstacle to action? Is a man more courageous if he fears much and nevertheless acts, or if he is relatively fearless? Several things must be said about this. In the first place it seems that the emotion of fear is not a necessary condition for the display of courage; in face of a great evil such as death or injury a man may show courage even if he does not tremble. On the other hand even irrational fears may give an occasion for courage: if someone suffers from claustrophobia or a dread of heights he may require courage to do that which would not be a courageous action for others. But not all fears belong from this point of view to the circumstances rather than to a man's character. For while we do not think of claustrophobia or a dread of heights as features of character, a general timorousness may be. Thus, although pathological fears are not the result of a man's choices and values some fears may be. The fears that count against a man's courage are those that we think he could overcome, and among them, in a special class, those that reflect the fact that he values safety too much.

In spite of problems such as these, which have certainly not all been solved, both the distinction between different kinds of obstacles to virtuous action and the general idea that virtues are correctives will be useful in resolving a difficulty in Kant's moral philosophy closely related to the issues discussed in the preceding paragraphs. In a passage in the first section of the *Groundwork of the Metaphysics of Morals* Kant notoriously tied himself into a knot in trying to give an account of those actions which have as he put it 'positive moral worth'. Arguing that only actions done out of a sense of duty have this worth he contrasts a philanthropist who 'takes pleasure in spreading happiness around him' with one who acts out of respect for duty, saying that the actions of the latter but not the former have moral worth. Much scorn has been poured on Kant for this curious doctrine, and indeed it does seem that something has gone wrong, but perhaps we are not in a position to scoff unless we can give our own account of the idea on which Kant is working. After all it does seem that he is right in saying that some actions are in accordance with duty, and even required by duty, without being the subjects of moral praise, like those of the honest trader who deals honestly in a situation in which it is in his interest to do so.

It was this kind of example that drove Kant to his strange conclusion. He added another example, however, in discussing acts of self-preservation; these he said, while they normally have no positive moral worth, may have it when a man preserves his life not from inclination but without inclination and from a sense of duty. Is he not right in saying that acts of self-preservation normally have no moral significance but that they may have it, and how do we ourselves explain this fact?

To anyone who approaches this topic from a consideration of the virtues the solution readily suggests itself. Some actions are in accordance with virtue without requiring virtue for their performance, whereas others are both in accordance with virtue and such as to show possession of a virtue. So Kant's trader was dealing honestly in a situation in which the virtue of honesty is not required for honest dealing, and it is for this reason that his action did not have 'positive moral worth'. Similarly, the care that one ordinarily takes for one's life, as for instance on some ordinary morning in eating one's breakfast and keeping out of the way of a car on the road, is something for which no virtue is required. As we said earlier there is no general virtue of self-love as there is a virtue of benevolence or charity, because men are generally attached sufficiently to their own good. Nevertheless in special circumstances virtues such as temperance, courage, fortitude, and hope may be needed if someone is to preserve his life. Are these circumstances in which the preservation of one's own life is a duty? Sometimes it is so, for sometimes it is what is owed to others that should keep a man from destroying himself, and then he may act out of a sense of duty. But not all cases in which acts of self-preservation show virtue are like this. For a man may display each of the virtues just listed even where he does not do any harm to others if he kills himself or fails to preserve his life. And it is this that explains why there may be a moral aspect to suicide which does not depend on possible injury to other people. It is not that suicide is 'always wrong', whatever that would mean, but that suicide is *sometimes* contrary to virtues such as courage and hope.

Let us now return to Kant's philanthropists, with the thought that it is action that is in accordance with virtue and also displays a virtue that has moral worth. We see at once that Kant's difficulties are avoided, and the happy philanthropist reinstated in the position which belongs to him. For charity is, as we said, a virtue of attachment as well as action, and the sympathy that makes it easier to act with charity is part of the virtue. The man who acts charitably out of a sense of duty is not to be undervalued, but it is the other who most shows virtue and therefore to the other that most moral worth is attributed. Only a detail of Kant's presentation of the case of the dutiful philanthropist tells on the other side. For what he actually said was that this man felt no sympathy and took no pleasure in the good of others because 'his mind was clouded by some sorrow of his own', and this is the kind of circumstance that increases the virtue that is needed if a man is to act well.

III

It was suggested above that an action with 'positive moral worth', or as we might say a positively good action, was to be seen as one which was in accordance with virtue, by which I mean contrary to no virtue, and moreover one for which a virtue was required. Nothing has so far been said about another case, excluded by the formula, in which it might seem that an act displaying one virtue was nevertheless contrary to another. In giving this last description I am thinking not of two virtues with competing claims, as if what were required by justice could nevertheless be demanded by charity, or something of that kind, but rather of the possibility that a virtue such as courage or temperance or industry which overcomes a special temptation, might be displayed in an act of folly or villainy. Is this something that we must allow for, or is it only good or innocent actions which can be acts of these virtues? Aquinas, in his definition of virtue, said that virtues can produce only good actions, and that they are dispositions 'of which no one can make bad use',[9] except when they are treated as objects, as in being the subject of hatred or pride. The common opinion nowadays is, however, quite different. With the notable exception of Peter Geach hardly anyone sees any difficulty in the thought that virtues may sometimes be displayed in bad actions. Von Wright, for instance, speaks of the courage of the villain as if this were a quite unproblematic idea, and most people take it for granted that the virtues of courage and temperance may aid a bad man in his evil work. It is also supposed that charity may lead a man to act badly, as when someone does what he has no right to do, but does it for the sake of a friend.

There are, however, reasons for thinking that the matter is not so simple as this. If a man who is willing to do an act of injustice to help a friend, or for the common good, is supposed to act out of charity, and he so acts where a just man will not, it should be said that the unjust man has more charity than the just man. But do we not think that someone not ready to act unjustly may yet be perfect in charity, the virtue having done its whole work in prompting him to do the acts that are permissible? And is there not more difficulty than might appear in the idea of an act of injustice which is nevertheless an act of courage? Suppose for instance that a sordid murder were in question, say a murder done for gain or to get an inconvenient person out of the way, but that this murder had to be done in alarming circumstances or in the face of real danger; should we be happy to say that such an action was an act of courage or a courageous act? Did the murderer, who certainly acted boldly, or with intrepidity, if he did the murder, also act courageously? Some people insist that they are ready to say this, but I have noticed that they like to move over to a murder for the sake of conscience, or to some other act done in the course of a villainous enterprise but whose immediate end is innocent or positively good. On their hypothesis, which is that bad acts can easily be seen as courageous acts or acts of courage, my original example should be just as good.

What are we to say about this difficult matter? There is no doubt that the murderer who murdered for gain was *not a coward*: he did not have a second moral defect which another villain might have had. There is no difficulty about this because it is clear that one defect may neutralise another. As Aquinas remarked, it is better for a blind horse if it is slow.[10] It does not follow, however, that an act of villainy can be courageous; we are inclined to say that it 'took courage', and yet it seems wrong to think of courage as equally connected with good actions and bad.

One way out of this difficulty might be to say that the man who is ready to pursue bad ends does indeed have courage, and shows courage in his action, but that in him courage is not a virtue. Later I shall consider some cases in which this might be the right thing to say, but in this instance it does not seem to be. For unless the murderer consistently pursues bad ends his courage will often result in good; it may enable him to do many innocent or positively good things for himself or for his family and friends. On the strength of an individual bad action we can hardly say that in him courage is not a virtue. Nevertheless there is something to be said even about the individual action to distinguish it from one that would readily be called an act of courage or a courageous act. Perhaps the following analogy may help us to see what it is. We might think of words such as 'courage' as naming characteristics of human beings in respect of a certain power, as words such as 'poison' and 'solvent' and 'corrosive' so name the properties of physical things. The power to which virtue-words are so related is the power of producing good action, and good desires. But just as poisons, solvents and corrosives do not always operate characteristically, so it could be with virtues. If P (say arsenic) is a poison it does not follow that P acts as a poison wherever it is found. It is quite natural to say on occasion 'P does not act as a poison here' though P is a poison and it is P that is acting here. Similarly courage is not operating as a virtue when the murderer turns his courage, which is a virtue, to bad ends. Not surprisingly the resistance that some of us registered was not to the expression 'the courage of the murderer' or to the assertion that what he did 'took courage' but rather to the description of that action as an act of courage or a courageous act. It is not that the action *could* not be so described, but that the fact that courage does not here have its characteristic operation is a reason for finding the description strange.

In this example we were considering an action in which courage was not operating as a virtue, without suggesting that in that agent it generally failed to do so. But the latter is also a possibility. If someone is both wicked and foolhardy this may be the case with courage, and it is even easier to find examples of a general connexion with evil rather than good in the case of some other virtues. Suppose, for instance, that we think of someone who is over-industrious, or too ready to refuse pleasure, and this is characteristic of him rather than something we find on one particular occasion. In this case the virtue of industry, or the virtue of temperance, has a systematic connexion with defective action rather than good action; and it might be said in either case that the virtue did not operate as a virtue in this man. Just as we might say in a certain setting 'P is not a poison here' though P is a poison and P is here, so we might say that industriousness, or temperance, is not a virtue in some. Similarly in a man habitually given to wishful thinking, who clings to false hopes, hope does not operate as a virtue and we may say that it is not a virtue in him.

The thought developed in the last paragraph, to the effect that not every man who has a virtue has something that is a virtue in him, may help to explain a certain discomfort that one may feel when discussing the virtues. It is not easy to put one's finger on what is wrong, but it has something to do with a disparity between the moral ideals that may seem to be implied in our talk about the virtues, and the moral judgements that we actually make. Someone reading the foregoing pages might, for instance, think that the author of this paper always admired most those people who had all the virtues, being wise and temperate as well as courageous, charitable, and just. And indeed it is sometimes so. There are some people who do possess all these virtues and who are loved and admired by all the world, as Pope John XXIII was loved and admired. Yet the fact is that many of us look up to some people whose chaotic lives contain rather little of wisdom or temperance, rather than to some others who possess these virtues. And while it may be that this is just romantic nonsense I suspect that it is not. For while wisdom always operates as a virtue, its close relation prudence does not, and it is prudence rather than wisdom that inspires many a careful life. Prudence is not a virtue in everyone, any more than industriousness is, for in some it is rather an over-anxious concern for safety and propriety, and a determination to keep away from people or situations which are apt to bring trouble with them; and by such defensiveness much good is lost. It is the same with temperance. Intemperance can be an appalling thing, as it was with Henry VIII of whom Wolsey remarked that

> rather than he will either miss or want any part of his will or appetite, he will put the loss of one half of his realm in danger.

Nevertheless in some people temperance is not a virtue, but is rather connected with timidity or with a grudging attitude to the acceptance of good things. Of course what is best is to live boldly yet without imprudence or intemperance, but the fact is that rather few can manage that.

Notes

1   G. H. von Wright, *The Varieties of Goodness* (London, 1963).
2   Peter Geach, *The Virtues* (Cambridge, 1977).
3   Aquinas, *Summa Theologica*, 1a2ae Q.56 a.3.
4   Aristotle, *Nicomachean Ethics*, especially bk. VII.
5   von Wright, *Varieties of Goodness*, chapter VIII.
6   Aristotle, *Nicomachean Ethics*, 1140 b 22–25. Aquinas, *Summa Theologica*, 1a2ae Q.57 a.4.
7   Aristotle, *Nicomachean Ethics*, 1106 b 15 and 1129 a.4 have this implication; but Aquinas is more explicit in *Summa Theologica*, 1a2ae Q.60 a.2.
8   Aquinas, *Summa Theologica*, 1a2ae Q.61 a.3.
9   Ibid., 1a2ae Q.56 a.5.
10 Ibid., 1a2ae Q.58 a.4.

5

Virtue and Reason

John McDowell

1. Presumably the point of, say, inculcating a moral outlook lies in a concern with how people live. It may seem that the very idea of a moral outlook makes room for, and requires, the existence of moral theory, conceived as a discipline which seeks to formulate acceptable principles of conduct. It is then natural to think of ethics as a branch of philosophy related to moral theory, so conceived, rather as the philosophy of science is related to science. On this view, the primary topic of ethics is the concept of right conduct, and the nature and justification of principles of behaviour. If there is a place for an interest in the concept of virtue, it is a secondary place. Virtue is a disposition (perhaps of a specially rational and self-conscious kind) to behave rightly; the nature of virtue is explained, as it were, from the outside in.

My aim is to sketch the outlines of a different view, to be found in the philosophical tradition which flowers in Aristotle's ethics. According to this different view, although the point of engaging in ethical reflections still lies in the interest of the question "How should one live?",[1] that question is necessarily approached *via* the notion of a virtuous person. A conception of right conduct is grasped, as it were, from the inside out.

2. I shall begin with some considerations which make it attractive to say, with Socrates, that virtue is knowledge.

What is it for someone to possess a virtue? "Knowledge" implies that he gets things right; if we are to go any distance towards finding plausibility in the Socratic thesis, it is necessary to start with examples whose status as virtues, and hence as states of character whose possessor arrives at right answers to a certain range of questions about how to

John McDowell, "Virtue and Reason," *Monist* (July 1979), 62(3): 331–50 (11).

behave, is not likely to be queried. I shall use the example of kindness; anyone who disputes its claim to be a virtue should substitute a better example of his own. (The objectivity which "knowledge" implies will recur later.)

A kind person can be relied on to behave kindly when that is what the situation requires. Moreover, his reliably kind behaviour is not the outcome of a blind, non-rational habit or instinct, like the courageous behaviour – so called only by courtesy – of a lioness defending her cubs.[2] Rather, that the situation requires a certain sort of behaviour is (one way of formulating) his reason for behaving in that way, on each of the relevant occasions. So it must be something of which, on each of the relevant occasions, he is aware. A kind person has a reliable sensitivity to a certain sort of requirement which situations impose on behaviour. The deliverances of a reliable sensitivity are cases of knowledge; and there are idioms according to which the sensitivity itself can appropriately be described as knowledge: a kind person knows what it is like to be confronted with a requirement of kindness. The sensitivity is, we might say, a sort of perceptual capacity.[3]

(Of course a kind person need not himself classify the behaviour he sees to be called for, on one of the relevant occasions, as kind. He need not be articulate enough to possess concepts of the particular virtues; and even if he does, the concepts need not enter his reasons for the actions which manifest those particular virtues. It is enough if he thinks of what he does, when – as we put it – he shows himself to be kind, under some such description as "the thing to do." The description need not differ from that under which he thinks of other actions of his, which we regard as manifesting different virtues; the division into actions which manifest kindness and actions which manifest other virtues can be imposed, not by the agent himself, but by a possibly more articulate, and more theoretically oriented, observer.)

The considerations adduced so far suggest that the knowledge constituted by the reliable sensitivity is a necessary condition for possession of the virtue. But they do not show that the knowledge is, as in the Socratic thesis, to be identified with the virtue. A preliminary case for the identification might go as follows. On each of the relevant occasions, the requirement imposed by the situation, and detected by the agent's sensitivity to such requirements, must exhaust his reason for acting as he does. It would disqualify an action from counting as a manifestation of kindness if its agent needed some extraneous incentive to compliance with the requirement – say, the rewards of a good reputation. So the deliverances of his sensitivity constitute, one by one, complete explanations of the actions which manifest the virtue. Hence, since the sensitivity fully accounts for its deliverances, the sensitivity fully accounts for the actions. But the concept of the virtue is the concept of a state whose possession accounts for the actions which manifest it. Since that explanatory role is filled by the sensitivity, the sensitivity turns out to be what the virtue is.[4]

That is a preliminary case for the identification of particular virtues with, as it were, specialized sensitivities to requirements. *Mutatis mutandis*, a similar argument applies to virtue in general. Indeed, in the context of another Socratic thesis, that of the unity of virtue, virtue in general is what the argument for identification with knowledge really concerns; the specialized sensitivities which are to be equated with particular virtues, according to the argument considered so far, are actually not available one by one for a series of separate identifications.

What makes this plausible is the attractive idea that a virtue issues in nothing but right conduct. Suppose the relevant range of behaviour, in the case of kindness, is marked out by the notion of proper attentiveness to others' feelings. Now sometimes acting in such a way as to indulge someone's feelings is not acting rightly: the morally important fact about the situation is not that A will be upset by a projected action (though he will), but, say, that B has a right – a consideration of a sort sensitivity to which might be thought of as constituting fairness. In such a case, a straightforward propensity to be gentle to others' feelings would not lead to right conduct. If a genuine virtue is to produce nothing but right conduct, a simple propensity to be gentle cannot be identified with the virtue of kindness. Possession of the virtue must involve not only sensitivity to facts about others' feelings as reasons for acting in certain ways, but also sensitivity to facts about rights as reasons for acting in certain ways; and when circumstances of both sorts obtain, and a circumstance of the second sort is the one that should be acted on, a possessor of the virtue of kindness must be able to tell that that is so.[5] So we cannot disentangle genuine possession of kindness from the sensitivity which constitutes fairness. And since there are obviously no limits on the possibilities for compresence, in the same situation, of circumstances of the sorts proper sensitivities to which constitute all the virtues, the argument can be generalized: no one virtue can be fully possessed except by a possessor of all of them, that is, a possessor of virtue in general. Thus the particular virtues are not a batch of independent sensitivities. Rather, we use the concepts of the particular virtues to mark similarities and dissimilarities among the manifestations of a single sensitivity which is what virtue, in general, is: an ability to recognize requirements which situations impose on one's behaviour. It is a single complex sensitivity of this sort which we are aiming to instil when we aim to inculcate a moral outlook.

3. There is an apparent obstacle to the identification of virtue with knowledge. The argument for the identification requires that the deliverances of the sensitivity – the particular pieces of knowledge with which it equips its possessor – should fully explain the actions which manifest virtue. But it is plausible that appropriate action need not be elicited by a consideration apprehended as a reason – even a conclusive reason – for acting in a certain way. That may seem to open the following possibility: a person's perception of a situation may precisely match what a virtuous person's perception of it would be, although he does not act as the virtuous person would. But if a perception which corresponds to the virtuous person's does not call forth a virtuous action from this non-virtuous person, then the virtuous person's matching perception – the deliverance of his sensitivity – cannot, after all, fully account for the virtuous action which it does elicit from him. Whatever is missing, in the case of the person who does not act virtuously, must be present as an extra component, over and above the deliverance of the sensitivity, in a complete specification of the reason why the virtuous person acts as he does.[6] That destroys the identification of virtue with the sensitivity. According to this line of argument, the sensitivity can be at most an ingredient in a composite state which is what virtue really is.

If we are to retain the identification of virtue with knowledge, then, by contraposition, we are committed to denying that a virtuous person's perception of a situation can be precisely matched in someone who, in that situation, acts otherwise than virtuously. Socrates seems to have supposed that the only way to embrace this commitment is in terms of ignorance, so that, paradoxically, failure to act as a virtuous person would cannot be voluntary, at least under that description. But there is a less extreme possibility, sketched by Aristotle.[7] This is to allow that someone who fails to act virtuously may, in a way, perceive what a virtuous person would, so that his failure to do the right thing is not inadvertent; but to insist that his failure occurs only because his appreciation of what he perceives is clouded, or unfocused, by the impact of a desire to do otherwise. This preserves the identification of virtue with a sensitivity; contrary to the counter-argument, nothing over and above the unclouded deliverances of the sensitivity is needed to explain the actions which manifest virtue. It is not that some extra explanatory factor, over and above the deliverances of the sensitivity, conspires with them to elicit action from the virtuous person, but rather that the other person's failure to act in that way is accounted for by a defectiveness in the approximations to those deliverances which he has.

It would be a mistake to protest that one can fail to act on a reason, and even on a reason judged by oneself to be better than any reason which one has for acting otherwise, without there needing to be any clouding or distortion in one's appreciation of the reason which one flouts.[8] That is true; but to suppose it constitutes an objection to Aristotle is to fail to understand the special nature of the conception of virtue which generates Aristotle's interest in incontinence.

One way to bring out the special nature of the conception is to note that, for Aristotle, continence is distinct from virtue, and just as problematic as incontinence. If someone needs to overcome an inclination to act otherwise, in getting himself to act as, say, temperance or courage demand, then he shows not virtue but (mere) continence. Suppose we take it that a virtuous person's judgment as to what he should do is arrived at by weighing, on the one side, some reason for acting in a way that will in fact manifest, say, courage, and, one the other side, a reason for doing something else (say a risk to life and limb, as a reason for running away), and deciding that on balance the former reason is the better. In that case, the distinction between virtue and continence will seem unintelligible. If the virtuous person allows himself to weigh the present danger, as a reason for running away, why should we not picture the weighing as his allowing himself to feel an inclination to run away, of a strength proportional to the weight which he allows to the reason? So long as he keeps the strength of his inclinations in line with the weight which he assigns to the reasons, his actions will conform to his judgment as to where, on balance, the better reason lies; what more can we require for virtue? (Perhaps that the genuinely courageous person simply does not care about his own survival? But Aristotle is rightly anxious to avert this misconception.[9]) The distinction becomes intelligible if we stop assuming that the virtuous person's judgment is a balancing of reasons for and against. The view of a situation which he arrives at by exercising his sensitivity is one in which some aspect of the situation is seen as constituting a reason for acting in some way; this reason is apprehended, not as outweighing or overriding any reasons for acting in other ways which would otherwise be constituted by other aspects of the situation (the present danger, say), but as silencing them. Here and now the risk to life and limb is not seen as any reason for removing himself. Aristotle's problem about incontinence is not "How can one weigh considerations in favour of actions X and Y, decide that on balance the better reasons are in favour of X, but nevertheless perform Y?" (a question which, no doubt, does not require the idea of clouded judgment for its answer); but rather (a problem equally about continence) "How can one have a view of a situation in which considerations which would otherwise appeal to one's will are silenced, but nevertheless allow those considerations to make themselves heard by one's will?" – a question which clearly is answerable, if at all, only by supposing that the incontinent or continent person does not fully share the virtuous person's perception of the situation.[10]

A more pressing objection is directed against the special conception of virtue: in particular, the use of cognitive notions in characterizing it. According to this objection, it must be a misuse of the notion of perception to suppose that an unclouded perception might suffice, on its own, to constitute a reason for acting in a certain way. An exercise of a genuinely cognitive capacity can yield at most part of a reason for acting; something appetitive is needed as well. To talk of virtue – a propensity to act in certain ways for certain reasons – as consisting in a sensitivity, a perceptual capacity, is to amalgamate the required appetitive component into the putative sensitivity. But all that is achieved thereby is a projection of human purposes into the world. (Here it becomes apparent how the objection touches on the issue of objectivity.) How one's will is disposed is a fact about oneself; whereas a genuinely cognitive faculty discloses to one how the world is independently of oneself, and in particular independently of one's will. Cognition and volition are distinct: the world – the proper sphere of cognitive capacities – is in itself an object of purely theoretical contemplation, capable of moving one to action only in conjunction with an extra factor – a state of will – contributed by oneself. I shall return to this objection.

4. Presented with an identification of virtue with knowledge, it is natural to ask for a formulation of the knowledge which virtue is. We tend to assume that the knowledge must have a stateable propositional content (perhaps not capable of immediate expression by the knower). Then the virtuous person's reliably right judgments as to what he should do, occasion by occasion, can be explained in terms of interaction between this universal knowledge and some appropriate piece of particular knowledge about the situation at hand; and the explanation can take the form of a "practical syllogism," with the content of the universal knowledge, or some suitable part of it, as major premiss, the relevant particular knowledge as minor premiss, and the judgment about what is to be done as deductive conclusion.

This picture is congenial to the objection mentioned at the end of §3. According to this picture, the problematic concept of a requirement figures only in the major premiss, and the conclusion, of the syllogism which reconstructs the virtuous person's reason for acting. Knowledge of the major premiss, the objector might say, is none other than the disposition of the will which is required, according to the objection, as a further component in the relevant reasons for acting, and hence as a further component in virtue, over and above any strictly cognitive state. (We call it "knowledge" to endorse it, not to indicate that it is genuinely cognitive.) What a virtuous person really perceives is only what is stated in the minor premiss of the syllogism: that is, a straightforward fact about the situation at hand, which – as the objection requires – would be incapable of eliciting action on its own.

This picture fits only if the virtuous person's views about how, in general, one should behave are susceptible of codification, in principles apt for serving as major premisses in syllogisms of the sort envisaged. But to an unprejudiced eye it should seem quite implausible that any reasonably adult moral outlook admits of any such codification. As Aristotle consistently says, the best generalizations about how one should behave hold only for the most part.[11] If one attempted to reduce one's conception of what virtue requires to a set of rules, then, however subtle and thoughtful one was in drawing up the code, cases would inevitably turn up in which a mechanical application of the rules would strike one as wrong – and not necessarily because one had changed one's mind; rather, one's mind on the matter was not susceptible of capture in any universal formula.[12]

A deep-rooted prejudice about rationality blocks ready acceptance of this. A moral outlook is a specific determination of one's practical rationality: it shapes one's views about what reasons one has for acting. Rationality requires consistency; a specific conception of rationality in a particular area imposes a specific form on the abstract requirement of consistency – a specific view of what counts as going on doing the same thing here. The prejudice is the idea that acting in the light of a specific conception of rationality must be explicable in terms of being guided by a formulable universal principle. This prejudice comes under radical attack in Wittgenstein's discussion, in the *Philosophical Investigations*, of the concept of following a rule.

Consider an exercise of rationality in which there *is* a formulable rule, of which each successive action can be regarded as an application, appropriate in the circumstances arrived at: say (Wittgenstein's example) the extending of a series of numbers. We tend to picture the understanding of the instruction "Add 2" – command of the rule for extending the series 2,4,6,8, . . . – as a psychological mechanism which, aside from lapses of attention and so forth, churns out the appropriate behaviour with the sort of reliability which a physical mechanism, say a piece of clockwork, might have. If someone is extending the series correctly, and one takes his behaviour to be compliance with the understood instruction, then, according to this picture, one has postulated such a psychological mechanism, underlying his behaviour, by an inference analogous to that whereby one might hypothesize a physical structure underlying the observable motions of some inanimate object. But this picture is profoundly suspect.

What manifests the pictured state of understanding? Suppose the person says, when asked what he is doing, "Look, I'm adding 2 each time." This apparent manifestation of understanding (or any other) will have been accompanied, at any point, by at most a finite fragment of the potentially infinite range of behaviour which we want to say the rule dictates. Thus the evidence for the presence of the pictured state is always compatible with the supposition that, on some future occasion for its exercise, the behaviour elicited by the occasion will diverge from what we would count as correct. Wittgenstein dramatizes this with the example of the man who continues the series, after 1000, with 1004, 1008, . . .[13] If a possibility of the 1004, 1008, . . . type were to be realized (and we could not bring the person to concede that he had simply made a mistake), that would show that the behaviour hitherto was not guided by the psychological conformation which we were picturing as guiding it. The pictured state, then, always transcends the grounds on which it is allegedly postulated.

There may be an inclination to protest: "This is merely inductive scepticism about other minds. After all, one knows in one's own case that one's behaviour will not come adrift like that." But this misses the point of the argument.

First, if what it is for one's behaviour to come adrift is for it suddenly to seem that everyone else is out of step, then clearly the argument bears on one's own case just as much as on the case of others. (Imagine that the person who goes on with 1004, 1008, . . . had said, in advance, "I know in my own case that my behaviour will not come adrift.")

Second, it is a mistake to interpret the argument as making a sceptical point: that one does not know, in the case of another person (or in one's own case either, once we have made the first correction), that the behaviour will not come adrift. The argument is not meant to suggest that we should be in a state of constant trepidation lest possibilities of the 1004,

1008, . . . type be realized.[14] We are confident that they will not: the argument aims, not at all to undermine this confidence, but to change our conception of its ground and nature. We tend to picture our transition to this confident expectation, from such grounds as we have, as being mediated by the postulated psychological mechanism. But we can no more find the putatively mediating state manifested in the grounds for our expectation than we can find manifested there the very future occurrences we expect. Postulation of the mediating state is an idle intervening step; it does nothing to underwrite the confidence of the expectation.

(The content of the expectation is not purely behavioural. We might have a good scientific argument, mediated by postulation of a physiological mechanism, for not expecting any particular train of behaviour, of the 1004, 1008, . . . type, which we might contemplate. Here postulation of the mediating physiological state would not be an idle intervening step. But the parallel is misleading. We can bring this out by considering a variant of Wittgenstein's example, in which, on reaching 1000, the person goes on as we expect, with 1002, 1004, . . . , but with a sense of dissociation from what he is doing. What he does no longer strikes him as going on in the same way; it feels as if a sheer habit has usurped his reason in controlling his behaviour. We confidently expect that this sort of thing will not happen; once again, postulation of a psychological mechanism does nothing to underwrite this confidence.)

What *is* the ground and nature of our confidence? About the competent use of words, Stanley Cavell writes:

> We learn and teach words in certain contexts, and then we are expected, and expect others, to be able to project them into further contexts. Nothing insures that this projection will take place (in particular, not the grasping of universals nor the grasping of books of rules), just as nothing insures that we will make, and understand, the same projections. That on the whole we do is a matter of our sharing routes of interest and feeling, modes of response, senses of humour and of significance and of fulfilment, of what is outrageous, of what is similar to what else, what a rebuke, what forgiveness, of when an utterance is an assertion, when an appeal, when an explanation – all the whirl of organism Wittgenstein calls "forms of life." Human speech and activity, sanity and community, rest upon nothing more, but nothing less, than this. It is a vision as simple as it is difficult, and as difficult as it is (and because it is) terrifying.[15]

The terror of which Cavell speaks at the end of this marvellous passage is a sort of vertigo, induced by the thought that there is nothing but shared forms of life to keep us, as it were, on the rails. We are inclined to think that is an insufficient foundation for a conviction that when we, say, extend a number series, we really are, at each stage, doing the same thing as before. In this mood, it seems to us that what Cavell describes cannot be a shared conceptual framework within which something is, given the circumstances, objectively the correct move;[16] it looks, rather, like a congruence of subjectivities, with the congruence not grounded as it would need to be to amount to an objectivity. So we feel we have lost the objectivity of (in our case) mathematics (and similarly in other cases). We recoil from this vertigo into the idea that we are kept on the rails by our grasp of rules. This idea has a pair of twin components: first, the idea (as above) that grasp of the rules is a psychological mechanism which (apart from mechanical failure, which is how we picture mistakes and so forth) guarantees that we stay in the straight and narrow; and, second, the idea that the rails – what we engage our mental wheels with when we come to grasp the rules – are objectively there, in a way which transcends the "mere" sharing of forms of life (hence, for instance, platonism about numbers). This composite idea is not the perception of some truth, but a consoling myth, elicited from us by our inability to endure the vertigo.

Of course, this casts no doubt on the possibility of putting explanations of particular moves, in the extending of a number series, in a syllogistic form: universal knowledge of how to extend the series interacts with particular knowledge of where one is in it, to produce a non-accidentally correct judgment as to what the next number is. In this case we can formulate the explanation so as to confer on the judgment explained the compellingness possessed by the conclusion of a proof. What is wrong is to take that fact to indicate that the explanation lays bare the inexorable workings of a machine: something whose operations, with our understanding of them, would not depend on the deliverances, in particular cases, of (for instance, and centrally) that shared sense of what is similar to what else which Cavell mentions. The truth is that it is only because of our own involvement in our "whirl of organism" that we can understand the words we produce as conferring that special compellingness on the judgment explained.

Now it is only this misconception of the deductive paradigm which leads us to suppose that the operations of any specific conception of rationality in a particular area – any specific conception of what counts as doing the same thing – must be deductively explicable; that is, that there must be a formulable universal principle suited to serve as major premiss in syllogistic explanations of the sort considered above.

Consider, for instance, a concept whose application gives rise to hard cases, in this sense: there are disagreements which resist resolution by argument, as to whether or not the concept applies. Convinced that one is in the right on a hard case, one will find oneself saying, as one's arguments tail off without securing assent, "You simply aren't seeing it," or "But don't you see?" In such cases the prejudice takes the form of a dilemma. One horn is that the inconclusiveness of one's arguments stems merely from an inability, in principle remediable, to articulate what one knows. It is possible, in principle, to spell out a universal formula which specifies the conditions under which the concept, in that use of it which one has mastered, is correctly applied. That would elevate one's argument to deductiveness. (If one's opponent refused to accept the deductive argument's major premiss, that would show that he had not mastered the same use of the concept, so that there would be, after all, no substantive disagreement.) If this assimilation to the deductive paradigm is not possible, then – this is the other horn of the dilemma – one's conviction that one is genuinely making a correct application of a concept (genuinely going on in the same way as before) must be an illusion. The case is revealed as one which calls, not for finding (seeing) the right answer to a question about how things are, but (perhaps) for a creative decision as to what to say.[17] Thus: either the case is not really a hard case, since sufficient ingenuity in the construction of arguments will resolve it; or, if its hardness is ineliminable, that shows that the issue cannot, after all, be one about whether an application of a concept is correct.

In a hard case, the issue turns on that appreciation of the particular instance whose absence is deplored, in "You simply aren't seeing it," or which is unsuccessfully appealed to, in "But don't you see?" The dilemma reflects the view that a putative judgment which is grounded in nothing firmer than that cannot really be going on in the same way as before. This is an avoidance of vertigo. The thought is: there is not enough there to constitute the rails on which a genuine series of consistent applications of a concept must run. But in fact it is an illusion to suppose that the first horn of the dilemma yields a way of preserving from risk of vertigo the conviction that we are dealing with genuine concept-application. The illusion is the misconception of the deductive paradigm: the idea that deductive explicability characterizes an exercise of reason in which it is, as it were, automatically compelling, without dependence on our partially shared "whirl of organism." The dilemma registers a refusal to accept that when the dependence which induces vertigo is out in the open, in the appeal to appreciation, we can genuinely be going on in the same way; but the paradigm of a genuine case, that with which the rejected case is unfavourably compared, has the same dependence, only less obviously.[18]

Contemplating the dependence should not induce vertigo at all. We cannot be whole-heartedly engaged in the relevant parts of the "whirl of organism," and at the same time achieve the detachment necessary in order to query whether our unreflective view of what we are doing is illusory. The cure for the vertigo, then, is to give up the idea that philosophical thought, about the sorts of practice in question, should be undertaken at some external standpoint, outside our immersion in our familiar forms of life.[19] If this cure works where explanations of exercises of rationality conform to the deductive paradigm, it should be no less efficacious where we explicitly appeal to appreciation of the particular instance in inviting acceptance of our judgments. And its efficacy in cases of the second kind is direct. Only the illusion that the deductive cases are immune can make it seem that, in order to effect the cure in cases of the second kind, we must first eliminate explicit dependence on appreciation, by assimilating them, as the prejudice requires, to the deductive paradigm.

If we make the assimilation, we adopt a position in which it is especially clear that our picture of a psychological mechanism, underlying a series of exercises of rationality, is a picture of something which transcends the grounds on which it is ascribed to anyone. In the cases in question, no one can express the envisaged universal formula. This transcendence poses difficulties about the acquisition of the pictured state. We are inclined to be impressed by the sparseness of the teaching which leaves someone capable of autonomously going on in the same way. All that happens is that the pupil is told, or shown, what to do in a few instances, with some surrounding talk about why that is the thing to do; the surrounding talk, *ex hypothesi* given that we are dealing with a case of the second kind, falls short of including actual enunciation of a universal principle, mechanical application of which would constitute correct behaviour in the practice in question. Yet pupils do acquire a capacity to go on, without further advice, to novel instances. Impressed by the sparseness of the teaching, we find this remarkable. But assimilation to the deductive paradigm leaves it no less remarkable. The assimilation replaces the question "How is it that the pupil, given that sparse instruction, goes on to new instances in the right way?" with the question "How is it that the pupil, given that sparse instruction, divines from it a universal formula with the right deductive powers?" The second question is, if anything, less tractable. Addressing the first, we can say: it is a fact (no doubt a remarkable fact) that, against a background of common human nature and shared forms of life, one's sensitivities to kinds of similarities between situations can be altered and enriched by just this sort of instruction. This attributes no guesswork to the learner; whereas no amount of appealing to common human nature and shared forms of life will free the second question from its presupposition – inevitably imported by assimilation to the deductive – that the learner is required to make a leap of divination.[20]

It is not to be supposed that the appreciation of the particular instance, explicitly appealed to in the second kind of case, is a straightforward or easy attainment on the part of those who have it; that either, on casual contemplation of an instance, one sees it in the right light, or else one does not, and is then unreachable by argument. First, "Don't you see?" can often be supplemented with words aimed at persuasion. A skifully presented characterization of an instance will sometimes bring someone to see it as one wants; or one can adduce general considerations, for instance about the point of the concept a particular application of which is in dispute. Given that the case is one of the second kind, any such arguments will fall short of rationally necessitating acceptance of their conclusion in the way a proof does.[21] But it is only the prejudice I am attacking which makes this seem to cast doubt on their status as arguments: that is, appeals to reason. Second, if effort can induce the needed appreciation in someone else, it can also take effort to acquire it oneself. Admitting the dependence on appreciation does not imply that, if someone has the sort of specific determination of rationality we are considering, the right way to handle a given situation will always be clear to him on unreflective inspection of it.

5. If we resist the prejudice, and respect Aristotle's belief that a view of how one should live is not codifiable, what happens to our explanations of a virtuous person's reliably right judgments as to what he should do on particular occasions? Aristotle's notion of the practical syllogism is obviously meant to apply here; we need to consider how.

The explanations, so far treated as explanations of judgments about what to do, are equally explanations of actions. The point of analogy which motivates the quasi-logical label "practical syllogism" is this. If something might serve as an argument for a theoretical conclusion, then it can equally figure in an account of someone's reasons for believing that conclusion, with the premisses of the argument giving the content of the psychological states – beliefs, in the theoretical case – which we cite in the reason-giving explanation. Now actions too are explained by reasons; that is, by citing psychological states in the light of which we can see how acting in the way explained would have struck the agent as in some way rational. The idea of a practical syllogism is the idea of an argument-like schema for explanations of actions, with the "premisses," as in the theoretical case, giving the content of the psychological states cited in the explanation.[22]

David Wiggins has given this account of the general shape of a practical syllogism:

> The first or major premiss mentions something of which there could be a desire, *orexis*, transmissible to some practical conclusion (i.e., a desire convertible *via* some available minor premiss into an action). The second premiss pertains to the feasibility in the particular situation to which the syllogism is applied of what must be done if the claim of the major premiss is to be heeded.[23]

This schema fits most straightforwardly when reasons are (in a broad sense) technical: the major premiss specifies a determinate goal, and the minor premiss marks out some action as a means to it.[24]

The role played by the major premiss, in these straightforward applications of the schema, is to give the content of an orectic psychological state: something we might conceive as providing the motivating energy for the actions explained. Aristotle's idea seems to be that what fills an analogous role in the explanation of virtuous actions is the virtuous person's conception of the sort of life a human being should lead.[25] If that conception were codifiable in universal principles, the explanations would take the deductive shape insisted on by the prejudice discussed in §4. But the thesis of uncodifiability means that the envisaged major premiss, in a virtue syllogism, cannot be definitively written down.[26] Any attempt to capture it in words will recapitulate the character of the teaching whereby it might be instilled: generalizations will be approximate at best, and examples will need to be taken with the sort of "and so on" which appeals to the cooperation of a hearer who has cottoned on.[27]

If someone guides his life by a certain conception of how to live, then he acts, on particular occasions, so as to fulfil suitable concerns.[28] A concern can mesh with a noticed fact about a situation, so as to account for an action: as, for instance, a concern for the welfare of one's friends, together with awareness that a friend is in trouble and open to being comforted, can explain missing a pleasant party in order to talk to the friend. On a suitable occasion, that pair of psychological states might constitute the core of a satisfying explanation of an action which is in fact virtuous. Nothing more need be mentioned for the action to have been given a completely intelligible motivation. In Aristotle's view, the orectic state cited in an explanation of a virtuous action is the agent's entire conception of how to live, rather than just whatever concern it happened to be; and this may now seem mysterious. But the core explanation, as so far envisaged, lacks any indication that the action explained conformed to the agent's conception of how to live. The core explanation would apply equally to a case of helping one's friend because one thought it was, in the circumstances, the thing to do, and to a case of helping one's friend in spite of thinking it was not, in the circumstances, the thing to do.

A conception of how one should live is not simply an unorganized collection of propensities to act, on this or that occasion, in pursuit of this or that concern. Sometimes there are several concerns, fulfilment of any one of which might, on a suitable occasion, constitute acting as a certain conception of how to live would dictate, and each of which, on the occasion at hand, is capable of engaging with a known fact about the situation and issuing in action. Acting in the light of a conception of how to live requires selecting and acting on the right concern. (Compare the end of §1, on the unity of virtue.) So if an action whose motivation is spelled out in our core explanation is a manifestation of virtue, more must be true of its agent than just that on this occasion he acted with that motivation. The core explanation must at least be seen against the background of the agent's conception of how to live; and if the situation is one of those on which any of several concerns might impinge, the conception of how to live must be capable of actually entering our understanding of the action, explaining why it was this concern rather than any other which was drawn into operation.

How does it enter? If the conception of how to live involved a ranking of concerns, or perhaps a set of rankings each relativized to some type of situation, the explanation of why one concern was operative rather than another would be straightforward. But uncodifiability rules out laying down such general rankings in advance of all the predicaments with which life may confront one.

What I have described as selecting the right concern might equally be described in terms of the minor premiss of the core explanation. If there is more than one concern which might impinge on the situation, there is more than one fact about the situation which the agent might, say, dwell on, in such a way as to summon an appropriate concern into operation. It is by virtue of his seeing this particular fact rather than that one as the salient fact about the situation that he is moved to act by this concern rather than that one.[29] This perception of saliences is the shape taken here by the appreciation of particular cases which I discussed in §5: something to which the uncodifiability of an exercise of rationality sometimes compels explicit appeal when we aim to represent actions as instances of it. A conception of how to live shows itself, when more than one concern might issue in action, in one's seeing, or being able to be brought to see, one fact rather than another as salient. And our understanding of such a conception enters into our understanding of actions – the supplementation which the core explanation needs – by enabling us to share, or at least comprehend, the agent's perception of saliences.[30]

It is not wrong to think of the virtuous person's judgments about what to do, or his actions, as explicable by interaction between knowledge of how to live and particular knowledge about the situation at hand. (Compare the beginning of §4.) But the thought needs a more subtle construal than the deductive paradigm allows. With the core explanations and their supplementations, I have in effect been treating the complete explanations as coming in two stages. It is at the first stage – hitherto the supplementation – that knowledge of how to live interacts with particular knowledge: knowledge, namely, of all the particular facts capable of engaging with concerns whose fulfilment would, on occasion, be virtuous. This interaction yields, in a way essentially dependent on appreciation of the particular case, a view of the situation with one such fact, as it were, in the foreground. Seen as salient, that fact serves, at the second stage, as minor premiss in a core explanation.[31]

6.   We can go back now to the non-cognitivist objection outlined at the end of §3. Awareness that one's friend is in trouble and open to being comforted – the psychological state whose content is the minor premiss of our core explanation – can perhaps, for the sake of argument, be conceded to be the sort of thing which the objection insists cognitive states must be: something capable of eliciting action only in conjunction with a non-cognitive state, namely, in our example, a concern for one's friends.[32] But if someone takes that fact to be the salient fact about the situation, he is in a psychological state which is essentially practical. The relevant notion of salience cannot be understood except in terms of seeing something as a reason for acting which silences all others (compare §3). So classifying that state as a cognitive state is just the sort of thing which the objection attacks.

The most natural way to press the objection is to insist on purifying the content of what is genuinely known down to something which is, in itself, motivationally inert (namely, given the concession above, that one's friend is in trouble and open to being comforted); and then to represent the "perception" of a salience as an amalgam of the purified awareness with an additional appetitive state. But what appetitive state? Concern for one's friends yields only the core explanation, not the explanation in which the "perception" of salience was to figure. Perhaps the conception of how to live? That is certainly an orectic state. But, given the thesis of uncodifiability, it is not intelligible independently of just such appreciation of particular situations as is involved in the present "perception" of a salience; so it is not suitable to serve as an element into which, together with some genuine awareness, the "perception" could be regarded as analysable. (This non-cognitivist strategy is reflected in assimilation to the deductive paradigm: that the assimilation is congenial to the non-cognitivist objection was noted early in §4. The failure of the strategy is reflected in the failure of the assimilation, given the thesis of uncodifiability.)

If we feel the vertigo discussed in §4, it is out of distaste for the idea that a manifestation of reason might be recognizable as such only from within the practice whose status is in question. We are inclined to think there ought to be a neutral external standpoint from which the rationality of any genuine exercise of reason could be demonstrated. Now we might understand the objection to be demanding a non-cognitive extra which would be analogous to hunger: an appetitive state whose possession by anyone is intelligible in its own right, not itself open to assessment as rational or irrational, but conferring an obvious rationality, recognizable from outside, on behaviour engaged in with a view to its gratification. In that case it is clear how the objection is an expression of the craving for a kind of rationality independently demonstrable as such. However, it is highly implausible that all the concerns which motivate virtuous actions are intelligible, one by one, independently of appreciating a virtuous person's distinctive way of seeing situations. And even if they were, the various particular concerns figure only in the core explanations. We do not fully understand a virtuous person's actions – we do not see the consistency in them – unless we can supplement the core explanations with a grasp of his conception of how to live. And though this is to credit him with an orectic state, it is not to credit him with an externally intelligible over-arching desire; for we cannot understand the content of the orectic state from the envisaged external standpoint. It is, rather, to comprehend, essentially from within, the virtuous person's distinctive way of viewing particular situations.[33]

The rationality of virtue, then, is not demonstrable from an external standpoint. But to suppose that it ought to be is only a version of the prejudice discussed in §4. It is only an illusion that our paradigm of reason, deductive argument, has its rationality discernible from a standpoint not necessarily located within the practice itself.

7.   Although perceptions of saliences resist decomposition into "pure" awareness together with appetitive states, there is an inclination to insist, nevertheless, that they cannot be genuinely cognitive states. We can be got into a cast of mind in which – as it seems to us – we have these problematic perceptions, only because we can be brought to care about certain things; hence, ultimately, only because of certain antecedent facts about our emotional and appetitive make-up. This can seem to justify a more subtle non-cognitivism: one which abandons the claim that the problematic perceptions can be analysed into cognitive and appetitive components, but insists that, because of the anthropocentricity of the conceptual apparatus involved, they are not judgments, true or false, as to how things are in an independent reality; and that is what cognitive states are.[34]

I cannot tackle this subtle non-cognitivism properly now. I suspect that its origin is a philistine scientism, probably based on the misleading idea that the right of scientific method to rational acceptance is discernible from a more objective standpoint than that from which we seem to perceive the saliences. A scientistic conception of reality is eminently open to dispute. When we ask the metaphysical question whether reality is what science can find out about, we cannot, without begging the question, restrict the materials for an answer to those which science can countenance. Let the question be an empirical question, by all means; but the empirical data which would be collected by a careful and sensitive moral phenomenology – no doubt not a scientific enterprise – are handled quite unsatisfyingly by non-cognitivism.[35]

It would be a mistake to object that stress on appreciation of the particular, and the absence of a decision procedure, encourages everyone to pontificate about particular cases. In fact resistance to non-cognitivism, about the perception of saliences, recommends humility. If we resist non-cognitivism, we can equate the conceptual equipment which forms the framework of anything recognizable as a moral outlook with a capacity to be impressed by certain aspects of reality. But ethical reality is immensely difficult to see clearly. (Compare the end of §4.) If we are aware of how, for instance, selfish fantasy distorts our vision, we shall not be inclined to be confident that we have got things right.[36]

It seems plausible that Plato's ethical Forms are, in part at least, a response to uncodifiability: if one cannot formulate what someone has come to know when he cottons on to a practice, say one of concept-application, it is natural to say that he has seen something. Now in the passage quoted in §4, Cavell mentions two ways of avoiding vertigo: "the grasping of universals" as well as what we have been concerned with so far, "the grasping of books of rules." But though Plato's Forms are a myth, they are not a consolation, a mere avoidance of vertigo; vision of them is portrayed as too difficult an attainment for that to be so. The remoteness of the Form of the Good is a metaphorical version of the thesis that value is not in the world, utterly distinct from the dreary literal version which has obsessed recent moral philosophy. The point of the metaphor is the colossal difficulty of attaining a capacity to cope clear-sightedly with the ethical reality which *is* part of our world. Unlike other philosophical responses to uncodifiability, this one may actually work towards moral improvement; negatively, by inducing humility, and positively, by an inspiring effect akin to that of a religious conversion.[37]

8. If the question "How should one live?" could be given a direct answer in universal terms, the concept of virtue would have only a secondary place in moral philosophy. But the thesis of uncodifiability excludes a head-on approach to the question whose urgency gives ethics its interest. Occasion by occasion, one knows what to do, if one does, not by applying universal principles but by being a certain kind of person: one who sees situations in a certain distinctive way. And there is no dislodging, from the central position they occupy in the ethical reflection of Plato and Aristotle, questions about the nature and (hardly discussed in this paper) the acquisition of virtue.

It is sometimes complained that Aristotle does not attempt to outline a decision procedure for questions about how to behave. But we have good reason to be suspicious of the assumption that there must be something to be found along the route he does not follow.[38] And there is plenty for us to do in the area of philosophy of mind where his different approach locates ethics.

Notes

1 Aristotle, *Nicomachean Ethics* (henceforth cited as *NE*), e.g., 1103b 26–31; cf. Plato, *Republic* 352d 5–6.

2 Cf. *NE* VI. 13 on the distinction between "natural virtue" and "virtue strictly so called."

3 Non-cognitivist objections to this sort of talk will be considered later.

4　There is a gap here. Even if it is conceded that the virtuous person has no further *reason* for what he does than the deliverance of his sensitivity, still, it may be said, two people can have the same reason for acting in a certain way, but only one of them act in that way. There must then be some further *explanation* of this difference between them: if not that the one who acts has a further reason, then perhaps that the one who does not is in some state, standing or temporary, which undermines the efficacy of reasons, or perhaps of reasons of the particular kind in question, in producing action. This suggests that if we are to think of virtue as guaranteeing action, virtue must consist not in the sensitivity alone but in the sensitivity together with freedom from such obstructive states. These issues recur in §3 below.

5　I do not mean to suggest that there is always a way of acting satisfactorily (as opposed to making the best of a bad job); nor that there is always one right answer to the question what one should do. But when there is a right answer, a virtuous person should be able to tell what it is.

6　If we distinguish the reason why he acts from his reason for acting, this is the objection of n4 above.

7　*NE* VII. 3.

8　Cf. Donald Davidson, "How is Weakness of Will Possible?," in Joel Feinberg, ed., *Moral Concepts* (Oxford: Oxford University Press, 1969), pp. 93–113, at pp. 99–100.

9　*NE* III. 9.

10　On this view, genuine deliverances of the sensitivity involved in virtue would necessitate action. It is not that action requires not only a deliverance of the sensitivity but also, say, freedom from possibly obstructive factors, for instance distracting desires. An obstructive factor would not interfere with the efficacy of a deliverance of the sensitivity, but rather preclude genuine achievement of that view of the situation. This fills the gap mentioned in n4 above. (My discussion of incontinence here is meant to do no more than suggest that the identification of virtue with knowledge should not be dismissed out of hand, on the ground that it poses a problem about incontinence. I have said a little more in §§9, 10 of my "Are Moral Requirements Hypothetical Imperatives?" *Proceedings of the Aristotelian Society Supplementary Volume 52* (1978), pp. 13–29; but a great deal more would be needed in a full treatment.)

11　See, e.g., *NE* I. 3.

12　See *NE* V. 10, especially 1137b 19–24.

13　*Philosophical Investigations* (Oxford: Basil Blackwell, 1953), §185.

14　Nor even that we really *understand* the supposition that such a thing might happen. See Barry Stroud, "Wittgenstein and Logical Necessity," *Philosophical Review* 74 (1965), pp. 504–18.

15　*Must We Mean What We Say?* (New York: Charles Scribner's Sons, 1969), p. 52.

16 Locating the desired objectivity *within* the conceptual framework is intended to leave open, here, the possibility of querying whether the conceptual framework itself is objectively the right one. If someone wants to reject the question whether this rather than that moral outlook is objectively correct, he will still want it to be an objective matter whether one has, say, succeeded in inculcating a particular moral outlook in someone else; so he will still be susceptible to the vertigo I am describing.

17 Why not abandon the whole practice as fraudulent? In some cases something may need to be said: for instance by a judge, in a lawsuit. Against the view that in legal hard cases judges are free to *make* the law, see Ronald Dworkin, "Hard Cases," in *Taking Rights Seriously* (London: Duckworth, 1977), pp. 81–130.

18 In the rejected case, the dependence is out in the open in an especially perturbing form, in that the occasional failure of the appeal to appreciation brings out how the "whirl of organism" is only partly shared; whereas there are no hard cases in mathematics. This is indeed a significant fact about mathematics. But its significance is not that mathematics is immune from the dependence.

19 I am not suggesting that effecting this cure is a simple matter.

20 See Wittgenstein, *Philosophical Investigations*, e.g., §210.

21 If general considerations recommend a universal formula, it will employ terms which themselves give rise to hard cases.

22 I distinguish practical reason from practical reasoning. From *NE* 1105a 28–33, with 1111a 15–16, it might seem that virtuous action, in Aristotle's view, must be the outcome of reasoning. But this doctrine is both incredible in itself and inconsistent with 1117a 17–22. So I construe Aristotle's discussion of deliberation as aimed at the reconstruction of reasons for action not necessarily thought out in advance; where they were not thought out in advance, the concept of deliberation applies in an "as if" style. See John M. Cooper, *Reason and Human Good in Aristotle* (Cambridge, Mass. and London: Harvard University Press, 1975), pp. 5–10. (It will be apparent that what I say about Aristotle's views on practical reason runs counter to Cooper's interpretation at many points. I am less concerned here with what Aristotle actually thought than with certain philosophical issues; so I have not encumbered this paper with scholarly controversy.)

23 David Wiggins, "Deliberation and Practical Reason," *Proceedings of the Aristotelian Society* 76 (1975–76): 29–51, at p. 40. The quoted passage is an explanation of Aristotle, *De Motu Animalium* 701a 9ff. My debt to Wiggins's paper will be apparent.

24 There is an inclination to insist on the only, or best, means. But this is the outcome of a suspect desire to have instances of the schema which *prove* that the action explained is the thing to do.

25 *NE* 1144a 31–3.

26 This is distinct from the claim that a person may at any stage be prone to change his mind (cf. §3 above). Wiggins (cited in n23 above) appears at some

points to run the two claims together, no doubt because he is concerned with practical reason generally, and not, as I am, with the expression in action of a specific conception of how to live. The line between realizing that one's antecedent conception of how to live requires something which one had not previously seen it to require, on the one hand, and modifying one's conception of how to live, on the other, is not a sharp one. But I do not want to exploit cases most happily described in the second way.

27   Cf. Wittgenstein, *Philosophical Investigations* §208.
28   I borrow this excellent term from Wiggins (cited in n23 above), p. 43ff.
29   This use of "salient" follows Wiggins, p. 45.
30   On the importance of the appreciation of the particular case, see *NE* 1142a 23–30, 1143a 25–b5; discussed by Wiggins, cited in n23, pp. 46–9. (For the point of "or at least comprehend", see n33 below.)
31   That the interaction, at the first stage, is with *all* the potentially reason-yielding facts about the situation allows us to register that, in the case of, say, courage, the gravity of the risk, in comparison to the importance of the end to be achieved by facing it, makes a difference to whether virtue really does require facing the risk; even though at the second stage, if the risk is not seen as salient, it is seen as no reason at all for running away. I am indebted here to a version of Wiggins's (cited in n23 above, p. 45), importantly modified for a revised excerpt from his paper in Joseph Raz, ed., *Practical Reasoning* (Oxford: Oxford University Press, 1978).
32   Actually this is open to question, because of special properties of the concept of a friend.
33   The qualification "essentially" is to allow for the possibility of appreciating what it is like to be inside a way of thinking without actually being inside it, on the basis of a sufficient affinity between it and a way of thinking of one's own. These considerations about externally intelligible desires bear on Philippa Foot's thesis, in "Morality as a System of Hypothetical Imperatives," *Philosophical Review* 81 (1972), pp. 305–16, that morality should be construed, or recast, in terms of hypothetical imperatives, on pain of being fraudulent. Her negative arguments seem to me to be analogous to an exposé of the emptiness of platonism, as affording a foundation for mathematical practice external to the practice itself. In the mathematical case it is not a correct response to look for another external guarantee of the rationality of the practice, but that seems to me just what Mrs Foot's positive suggestion amounts to in the moral case. (If the desires are not externally intelligible the label "hypothetical imperative" loses its point.) See, further, my "Are Moral Requirements Hypothetical Imperatives?" cited in n10 above.
34   On anthropocentricity, see David Wiggins, "Truth, Invention, and the Meaning of Life," *Proceedings of the British Academy* 62 (1976), 331–78, at pp. 348–9, 360–3.
35   See Wiggins, cited in n34, above; and Iris Murdoch, *The Sovereignty of Good* (London: Routledge and Kegan Paul, 1970).

36 Cf. Iris Murdoch, cited n35, above. I am indebted here to Mark Platts.
37 This view of Plato is beautifully elaborated by Iris Murdoch.
38 The idea, for instance, that something like utilitarianism *must* be right looks like a double avoidance of vertigo: first, in the thought that there must be a decision procedure; and second, in the reduction of practical rationality to the pursuit of neutrally intelligible desires.

The Nature of the Virtues

Alasdair MacIntyre

One response to the history which I have narrated so far might well be to suggest that even within the relatively coherent tradition of thought which I have sketched there are just too many different and incompatible conceptions of a virtue for there to be any real unity to the concept or indeed to the history. Homer, Sophocles, Aristotle, the New Testament and medieval thinkers differ from each other in too many ways. They offer us different and incompatible lists of the virtues; they give a different rank order of importance to different virtues; and they have different and incompatible theories of the virtues. If we were to consider later Western writers on the virtues, the list of differences and incompatibilities would be enlarged still further; and if we extended our enquiry to Japanese, say, or American Indian cultures, the differences would become greater still. It would be all too easy to conclude that there are a number of rival and alternative conceptions of the virtues, but, even within the tradition which I have been delineating, no single core conception.

The case for such a conclusion could not be better constructed than by beginning from a consideration of the very different lists of items which different authors in different times and places have included in their catalogues of virtues. Some of these catalogues – Homer's, Aristotle's and the New Testament's – I have already noticed at greater or lesser length. Let me at the risk of some repetition recall some of their key features and then introduce for further comparison the catalogues of two later Western writers, Benjamin Franklin and Jane Austen.

The first example is that of Homer. At least some of the items in a Homeric list of the *aretai* would clearly not be counted by most of us

Alasdair MacIntyre, "The Nature of the Virtues," *After Virtue* (London: Duckworth, 1985), pp. 169–89.

nowadays as virtues at all, physical strength being the most obvious example. To this it might be replied that perhaps we ought not to translate the word *aretê* in Homer by our word 'virtue', but instead by our word 'excellence'; and perhaps, if we were so to translate it, the apparently surprising difference between Homer and ourselves would at first sight have been removed. For we could allow without any kind of oddity that the possession of physical strength is the possession of an excellence. But in fact we would not have removed, but instead would merely have relocated, the difference between Homer and ourselves. For we would now seem to be saying that Homer's concept of an *aretê*, an excellence, is one thing and that our concept of a virtue is quite another since a particular quality can be an excellence in Homer's eyes, but not a virtue in ours and *vice versa*.

But of course it is not that Homer's list of virtues differs only from our own; it also notably differs from Aristotle's. And Aristotle's of course also differs from our own. For one thing, as I noticed earlier, some Greek virtue-words are not easily translatable into English or rather out of Greek. Moreover consider the importance of friendship as a virtue in Aristotle's list – how different from us! Or the place of *phronêsis* – how different from Homer and from us! The mind receives from Aristotle the kind of tribute which the body receives from Homer. But it is not just the case that the difference between Aristotle and Homer lies in the inclusion of some items and the omission of others in their respective catalogues. It turns out also in the way in which those catalogues are ordered, in which items are ranked as relatively central to human excellence and which marginal.

Moreover the relationship of virtues to the social order has changed. For Homer the paradigm of human excellence is the warrior; for Aristotle it is the Athenian gentleman. Indeed according to Aristotle certain virtues are only available to those of great riches and of high social status; there are virtues which are unavailable to the poor man, even if he is a free man. And those virtues are on Aristotle's view ones central to human life; magnanimity – and once again, any translation of *megalopsuchia* is unsatisfactory – and munificence are not just virtues, but important virtues within the Aristotelian scheme.

At once it is impossible to delay the remark that the most striking contrast with Aristotle's catalogue is to be found neither in Homer's nor in our own, but in the New Testament's. For the New Testament not only praises virtues of which Aristotle knows nothing – faith, hope and love – and says nothing about virtues such as *phronêsis* which are crucial for Aristotle, but it praises at least one quality as a virtue which Aristotle seems to count as one of the vices relative to magnanimity, namely humility. Moreover since the New Testament quite clearly sees the rich as destined for the pains of Hell, it is clear that the key virtues cannot be available to them; yet they *are* available to slaves. And the New Testament of course differs from both Homer and Aristotle not only in the items included in its catalogue, but once again in its rank ordering of the virtues.

Turn now to compare all three lists of virtues considered so far – the Homeric, the Aristotelian, and the New Testament's – with two much later lists, one which can be compiled from Jane Austen's novels and the other which Benjamin Franklin constructed for himself. Two features stand out in Jane Austen's list. The first is the importance that she allots to the virtue which she calls 'constancy', a virtue about which I say more [in a later chapter]. In some ways constancy plays a role in Jane Austen analogous to that of *phronêsis* is Aristotle; it is a virtue the possession of which is a prerequisite for the possession of other virtues. The second is the fact that what Aristotle treats as the virtue of agreeableness (a virtue for which he says there is no name) she treats as only the simulacrum of a genuine virtue – the genuine virtue in question is the one she calls amiability. For the man who practices agreeableness does so from considerations of honour and expediency, according to Aristotle; whereas Jane Austen thought it possible and necessary for the possessor of that virtue to have a certain real affection for people as such. (It matters here that Jane Austen is a Christian.) Remember that Aristotle himself had treated military courage as a simulacrum of true courage. Thus we find here yet another type of disagreement over the virtues; namely, one as to which human qualities are genuine virtues and which mere simulacra.

In Benjamin Franklin's list we find almost all the types of difference from at least one of the other catalogues we have considered and one more. Franklin includes virtues which are new to our consideration such as cleanliness, silence and industry; he clearly considers the drive to acquire itself a part of virtue, whereas for most ancient Greeks this is the vice of *pleonexia*; he treats some virtues which earlier ages had considered minor as major; but he also redefines some familiar virtues. In the list of thirteen virtues which Franklin compiled as part of his system of private moral accounting, he elucidates each virtue by citing a maxim obedience to which *is* the virtue in question. In the case of chastity the maxim is 'Rarely use venery but for health or offspring – never to dullness, weakness or the injury of your own or another's peace or reputation'. This is clearly not what earlier writers had meant by 'chastity'.

We have therefore accumulated a startling number of differences and incompatibilities in the five stated and implied accounts of the virtues. So the question which I raised at the outset becomes more urgent. If different writers in different times and places, but all within the history of Western culture, include such different sets and types of items in their lists, what grounds have we for supposing that they do indeed aspire to list items of one and the same kind, that there is any shared concept at all? A second kind of consideration reinforces the presumption of a negative answer to this question. It is not just that each of these five writers lists different and differing kinds of items; it is also that each of these lists embodies, is the expression of a different theory about what a virtue is.

In the Homeric poems a virtue is a quality the manifestation of which enables someone to do exactly what their well-defined social role requires. The primary role is that of the warrior king and that Homer lists those virtues which he does becomes intelligible at once when we recognise that the key virtues therefore must be those which enable a man to excel in combat and in the games. It follows that we cannot identify the Homeric virtues until we have first identified the key social roles in Homeric society and the requirements of each of them. The concept of *what anyone filling such-and-such a role ought to do* is prior to the concept of a virtue; the latter concept has application only via the former.

On Aristotle's account matters are very different. Even though some virtues are available only to certain types of people, none the less virtues attach not to men as inhabiting social roles, but to man as such. It is the *telos* of man as a species which determines what human qualities are virtues. We need to remember however that although Aristotle treats the acquisition and exercise of the virtues as means to an end, the relationship of means to end is internal and not external. I call a means internal to a given end when the end cannot be adequately characterised independently of a characterisation of the means. So it is with the virtues and the *telos* which is the good life for man on Aristotle's account. The exercise of the virtues is itself a crucial component of the good life for man. This distinction between internal and external means to an end is not drawn by Aristotle himself in the *Nicomachean Ethics*, as I noticed earlier, but it is an essential distinction to be drawn if we are to understand what Aristotle intended. The distinction *is* drawn explicitly by Aquinas in the course of his defence of St Augustine's definition of a virtue, and it is clear that Aquinas understood that in drawing it he was maintaining an Aristotelian point of view.

The New Testament's account of the virtues, even if it differs as much as it does in content from Aristotle's – Aristotle would certainly not have admired Jesus Christ and he would have been horrified by St Paul – does have the same logical and conceptual structure as Aristotle's account. A virtue is, as with Aristotle, a quality the exercise of which leads to the achievement of the human *telos*. *The* good for man is of course a supernatural and not only a natural good, but supernature redeems and completes nature. Moreover the relationship of virtues as means to the end which is human incorporation in the divine kingdom of the age to come is internal and not external, just as it is in Aristotle. It is of course this parallelism which allows Aquinas to synthesise Aristotle and the New Testament. A key feature of this parallelism is the way in which the concept of *the good life for man* is prior to the concept of a virtue in just the way in which on the Homeric account the concept of a social role was prior. Once again it is the way in which the former concept is applied which determines how the latter is to be applied. In both cases the concept of a virtue is a secondary concept.

The intent of Jane Austen's theory of the virtues is of another kind. C. S. Lewis has rightly emphasised how profoundly Christian her moral vision is and Gilbert Ryle has equally rightly emphasised her inheritance from Shaftesbury and from Aristotle. In fact her views combine elements from Homer as well, since she is concerned with social roles in a way that neither the New Testament nor Aristotle are. She is therefore important for the way in which she finds it possible to combine what are at first sight disparate theoretical accounts of the virtues. But for the moment any attempt to assess the significance of Jane Austen's synthesis must be delayed. Instead we must notice the quite different style of theory articulated in Benjamin Franklin's account of the virtues.

Franklin's account, like Aristotle's, is teleological; but unlike Aristotle's, it is utilitarian. According to Franklin in his *Autobiography* the virtues are means to an end, but he envisages the means–ends relationship as external rather than internal. The end to which the cultivation of the virtues ministers is happiness, but happiness understood as success, prosperity in Philadelphia and ultimately in heaven. The virtues are to be useful and Franklin's account continuously stresses utility as a criterion in individual cases: 'Make no expence but to do good to others or yourself; i.e. waste nothing', 'Speak not but what may benefit others or yourself. Avoid trifling conversation' and, as we have already seen, 'Rarely use venery but for health or offspring . . .' When Franklin was in Paris he was horrified by Parisian architecture: 'Marble, porcelain and gilt are squandered without utility.'

We thus have at least three very different conceptions of a virtue to confront: a virtue is a quality which enables an individual to discharge his or her social role (Homer); a virtue is a quality which enables an individual to move towards the achievement of the specifically human *telos*, whether natural or supernatural (Aristotle, the New Testament and Aquinas); a virtue is a quality which has utility in achieving earthly and heavenly success (Franklin). Are we to take these as three rival accounts of the same thing? Or are they instead accounts of three different things? Perhaps the moral structures in archaic Greece, in fourth-century Greece, and in eighteenth-century Pennsylvania were so different from each other that we should treat them as embodying quite different concepts, whose difference is initially disguised from us by the historical accident of an inherited vocabulary which misleads us by linguistic resemblance long after conceptual identity and similarity have failed. Our initial question has come back to us with redoubled force.

Yet although I have dwelt upon the *prima facie* case for holding that the differences and incompatibilities between different accounts at least suggest that there is no single, central, core conception of the virtues which might make a claim for universal allegiance, I ought also to point out that each of the five moral accounts which I have sketched so summarily does embody just such a claim. It is indeed just this feature of those accounts that makes them of more than sociological or antiquarian interest. Every one of these accounts claims not only theoretical, but also an institutional hegemony. For Odysseus the Cyclopes stand condemned because they lack agriculture, on *agora* and *themis*. For Aristotle the barbarians stand condemned because they lack the *polis* and are therefore incapable of politics. For New Testament Christians there is no salvation outside the apostolic church. And we know that Benjamin Franklin found the virtues more at home in Philadelphia than in Paris and that for Jane Austen the touchstone of the virtues is a certain kind of marriage and indeed a certain kind of naval officer (that is, a certain kind of *English* naval officer).

The question can therefore now be posed directly: are we or are we not able to disentangle from these rival and various claims a unitary core concept of the virtues of which we can give a more compelling account than any of the other accounts so far? I am going to argue that we can in fact discover such a core concept and that it turns out to provide the tradition of which I have written the history with its conceptual unity. It will indeed enable us to distinguish in a clear way those beliefs about the virtues which genuinely belong to the tradition from those which do not. Unsurprisingly perhaps it is a complex concept, different parts of which derive from different stages in the development of the tradition. Thus the concept itself in some sense embodies the history of which it is the outcome.

One of the features of the concept of a virtue which has emerged with some clarity from the argument so far is that it always requires for its application the acceptance of some prior account of certain features of social and moral life in terms of which it has to be defined and explained. So in the Homeric account the concept of a virtue is secondary to that of *a social role*, in Aristotle's account it is secondary to that of *the good life for man* conceived as the *telos* of human action and in Franklin's much later account it is secondary to that of utility. What is it in the account which I am about to give which provides in a similar way the necessary background against which the concept of a virtue has to be made intelligible? It is in answering this question that the complex, historical, multilayered character of the core concept of virtue becomes clear. For there are no less than three stages in the logical development of the concept which have to be identified in order, if the core conception of a virtue is to be understood, and each of these stages has its own conceptual background. The first stage requires a background account of what I shall call a practice, the second an account of what I have already characterised as the narrative order of a single human life and the third an account a good deal fuller than I have given up to now of what constitutes a moral tradition. Each later stage presupposes the earlier, but not *vice versa*. Each earlier stage is both modified by and reinterpreted in the light of, but also provides an essential constituent of each later stage. The progress in the development of the concept is closely related to, although it does not recapitulate in any straightforward way, the history of the tradition of which it forms the core.

In the Homeric account of the virtues – and in heroic societies more generally – the exercise of a virtue exhibits qualities which are required for sustaining a social role and for exhibiting excellence in some well-marked area of social practice: to excel is to excel at war or in the games, as Achilles does, in sustaining a household, as Penelope does, in giving counsel in the assembly, as Nestor does, in the telling of a tale, as Homer himself does. When Aristotle speaks of excellence in human activity, he sometimes though not always, refers to some well-defined type of human practice: flute-playing, or war, or geometry. I am going to suggest that this notion of a particular type of practice as providing the arena in which the virtues are exhibited and in terms of which they are to receive their primary, if incomplete, definition is crucial to the whole enterprise of identifying a core concept of the virtues. I hasten to add two *caveats* however.

The first is to point out that my argument will not in any way imply that virtues are *only* exercised in the course of what I am calling practices.

The second is to warn that I shall be using the word 'practice' in a specially defined way which does not completely agree with current ordinary usage, including my own previous use of that word. What am I going to mean by it?

By a 'practice' I am going to mean any coherent and complex form of socially established cooperative human activity through which goods internal to that form of activity are realised in the course of trying to achieve those standards of excellence which are appropriate to, and partially definitive of, that form of activity, with the result that human powers to achieve excellence, and human conceptions of the ends and goods involved, are systematically extended. Tic-tac-toe is not an example of a practice in this sense, nor is throwing a football with skill; but the game of football is, and so is chess. Bricklaying is not a practice; architecture is. Planting turnips is not a practice; farming is. So are the enquiries of physics, chemistry and biology, and so is the work of the historian, and so are painting and music. In the ancient and medieval worlds the creation and sustaining of human communities – of households, cities, nations – is generally taken to be a practice in the sense in which I have defined it. Thus the range of practices is wide: arts, sciences, games, politics in the Aristotelian sense, the making and sustaining of family life, all fall under the concept. But the question of the precise range of practices is not at this stage of the first importance. Instead let me explain some of the key terms involved in my definition, beginning with the notion of goods internal to a practice.

Consider the example of a highly intelligent seven-year-old child whom I wish to teach to play chess, although the child has no particular desire to learn the game. The child does however have a very strong desire for candy and little chance of obtaining it. I therefore tell the child that if the child will play chess with me once a week I will give the child 50¢ worth of candy; moreover I tell the child that I will always play in such a way that it will be difficult, but not impossible, for the child to win and that, if the child wins, the child will receive an extra 50¢ worth of candy. Thus motivated the child plays and plays to win. Notice however that, so long as it is the candy alone which provides the child with a good reason for playing chess, the child has no reason not to cheat and every reason to cheat, provided he or she can do so successfully. But, so we may hope, there will come a time when the child will find in those goods specific to chess, in the achievement of a certain highly particular kind of analytical skill, strategic imagination and competitive intensity, a new set of reasons, reasons now not just for winning on a particular occasion, but for trying to excel in whatever way the game of chess demands. Now if the child cheats, he or she will be defeating not me, but himself or herself.

There are thus two kinds of good possibly to be gained by playing chess. On the one hand there are those goods externally and contingently attached to chess-playing and to other practices by the accidents of social circumstance – in the case of the imaginary child candy, in the case of real adults such goods as prestige, status and money. There are always alternative ways for achieving such goods, and their achievement is never to be had *only* by engaging in some particular kind of practice. On the other hand there are the goods internal to the practice of chess which cannot be had in any way but by playing chess or some other game of that specific kind. We call them internal for two reasons: first, as I have already suggested, because we can only specify them in terms of chess or some other game of that specific kind and by means of examples from such games (otherwise the meagerness of our vocabulary for speaking of such goods forces us into such devices as my own resort to writing of 'a certain highly particular kind of'); and secondly because they can only be identified and recognised by the experience of participating in the practice in question. Those who lack the relevant experience are incompetent thereby as judges of internal goods.

This is clearly the case with all the major examples of practices: consider for example – even if briefly and inadequately – the practice of portrait painting as it developed in Western Europe from the late middle ages to the eighteenth century. The successful portrait painter is able to achieve many goods which are in the sense just defined external to the practice of portrait painting – fame, wealth, social status, even a measure of power and influence at courts upon occasion. But those external goods are not to be confused with the goods which are internal to the practice. The internal goods are those which result from an extended attempt to show how Wittgenstein's dictum 'The human body is the best picture of the human soul' (*Investigations*, p. 178e) might be made to become true by teaching us 'to regard . . . the picture on our wall as the object itself (the men, landscape and so on) depicted there' (p. 205e) in a quite new way. What is misleading about Wittgenstein's dictum as it stands is its neglect of the truth in George Orwell's thesis 'At 50 everyone has the face he deserves'. What painters from Giotto to Rembrandt learnt to show was how the face at any age may be revealed as the face that the subject of a portrait deserves.

Originally in medieval paintings of the saints the face was an icon; the question of a resemblance between the depicted face of Christ or St Peter and the face that Jesus or Peter actually possessed at some particular age did not even arise. The antithesis to this iconography was the relative naturalism of certain fifteenth-century Flemish and German painting. The heavy eyelids, the coifed hair, the lines around the mouth undeniably represent some particular woman, either actual or envisaged. Resemblance has usurped the iconic relationship. But with Rembrandt there is, so to speak, synthesis: the naturalistic portrait is now rendered as an icon, but an icon of a new and hitherto inconceivable kind. Similarly in a very different kind of sequence mythological faces in a certain kind of seventeenth-century French painting become aristocratic faces in the eighteenth century. Within each of these sequences at least two different kinds of good internal to the painting of human faces and bodies are achieved.

There is first of all the excellence of the products, both the excellence in performance by the painters and that of each portrait itself. This excellence – the very verb 'excel' suggests it – has to be understood historically. The sequences of development find their point and purpose in a progress towards and beyond a variety of types and modes of excellence. There are of course sequences of decline as well as of progress, and progress is rarely to be understood as straightforwardly linear. But it is in participation in the attempts to sustain progress and to respond creatively to moments that the second kind of good internal to the practices of portrait painting is to be found. For what the artist discovers within the pursuit of excellence in portrait painting – and what is true of portrait painting is true of the practice of the fine arts in general – is the good of a certain kind of life. That life may not constitute the whole of life for someone who is a painter by a very long way or it may at least for a period, Gauguin-like, absorb him or her at the expense of almost everything else. But it is the painter's living out of a greater or lesser part of his or her life *as a painter* that is the second kind of good internal to painting. And judgment upon these goods requires at the very least the kind of competence that is only to be acquired either as a painter or as someone willing to learn systematically what the portrait painter has to teach.

A practice involves standards of excellence and obedience to rules as well as the achievement of goods. To enter into a practice is to accept the authority of those standards and the inadequacy of my own performance as judged by them. It is to subject my own attitudes, choices, preferences and tastes to the standards which currently and partially define the practice. Practices of course, as I have just noticed, have a history: games, sciences and arts all have histories. Thus the standards are not themselves immune from criticism, but none the less we cannot be initiated into a practice without accepting the authority of the best standards realised so far. If, on starting to listen to music, I do not accept my own incapacity to judge correctly, I will never learn to hear, let alone to appreciate, Bartok's last quartets. If, on starting to play baseball, I do not accept that others know better than I when to throw a fast ball and when not, I will never learn to appreciate good pitching let alone to pitch. In the realm of practices the authority of both goods and standards operates in such a way as to rule out all subjectivist and emotivist analyses of judgment. De gustibus *est* disputandum.

We are now in a position to notice an important difference between what I have called internal and what I have called external goods. It is characteristic of what I have called external goods that when achieved they are always some individual's property and possession. Moreover characteristically they are such that the more someone has of them, the less there is for other people. This is sometimes necessarily the case, as with power and fame, and sometimes the case by reason of contingent circumstance as with money. External goods are therefore characteristically objects of competition in which there must be losers as well as winners. Internal goods are indeed the outcome of competition to excel, but it is characteristic of them that their achievement is a good for the whole community who participate in the practice. So when Turner transformed the seascape in painting or W. G. Grace advanced the art of batting in cricket in a quite new way their achievement enriched the whole relevant community.

But what does all or any of this have to do with the concept of the virtues? It turns out that we are now in a position to formulate a first, even if partial and tentative definition of a virtue: *A virtue is an acquired human quality the possession and exercise of which tends to enable us to achieve those goods which are internal to practices and the lack of which effectively prevents us from achieving any such goods.* Later this definition will need amplification and amendment. But as a first approximation to an adequate definition it already illuminates the place of the virtues in human life. For it is not difficult to show for a whole range of key virtues that without them the goods internal to practices are barred to us, but not just barred to us generally, barred in a very particular way.

It belongs to the concept of a practice as I have outlined it – and as we are all familiar with it already in our actual lives, whether we are painters or physicists or quarterbacks or indeed just lovers of good painting or first-rate experiments or a well-thrown pass – that its goods can only be achieved by subordinating ourselves to the best standard so far achieved, and that entails subordinating ourselves within the practice in our relationship to other practitioners. We have to learn to recognise what is due to whom; we have to be prepared to take whatever self-endangering risks are demanded along the way; and we have to listen carefully to what we are told about our own inadequacies and to reply with the same carefulness for the facts. In other words we have to accept as necessary components of any practice with internal goods and standards of excellence the virtues of justice, courage and honesty. For not to accept these, to be willing to cheat as our imagined child was willing to cheat in his or her early days at chess, so far bars us from achieving the standards of excellence or the goods internal to the practice that it renders the practice pointless except as a device for achieving external goods.

We can put the same point in another way. Every practice requires a certain kind of relationship between those who participate in it. Now the virtues are those goods by reference to which, whether we like it or not, we define our relationships to those other people with whom we share the kind of purposes and standards which inform practices. Consider an example of how reference to the virtues has to be made in certain kinds of human relationship.

A, B, C, and D are friends in that sense of friendship which Aristotle takes to be primary: they share in the pursuit of certain goods. In my terms they share in a practice. D dies in obscure circumstances, A discovers how D died and tells the truth about it to B while lying to C. C discovers the lie. What A cannot then intelligibly claim is that he stands in the same relationship of friendship to both B and C. By telling the truth to one and lying to the other he has partially defined a difference in the relationship. Of course it is open to A to explain this difference in a number of ways; perhaps he was trying to spare C pain or perhaps he is simply cheating C. But some difference in the relationship now exists as a result of the lie. For their allegiance to each other in the pursuit of common goods has been put in question.

Just as, so long as we share the standards and purposes characteristic of practices, we define our relationships to each other, whether we acknowledge it or not, by reference to standards of truthfulness and trust, so we define them too by reference to standards of justice and of courage. If A, a professor, gives B and C the grades that their papers deserve, but grades D because he is attracted by D's blue eyes or is repelled by D's dandruff, he has defined his relationship to D differently from his relationship to the other members of the class, whether he wishes it or not. Justice requires that we treat others in respect of merit or desert according to uniform and impersonal standards; to depart from the standards of justice in some particular instance defines our relationship with the relevant person as in some way special or distinctive.

The case with courage is a little different. We hold courage to be a virtue because the care and concern for individuals, communities and causes which is so crucial to so much in practices requires the existence of such a virtue. If someone says that he cares for some individual, community or cause, but is unwilling to risk harm or danger on his, her or its own behalf, he puts in question the genuineness of his care and concern. Courage, the capacity to risk harm or danger to oneself, has its role in human life because of this connection with care and concern. This is not to say that a man cannot genuinely care and also be a coward. It is in part to say that a man who genuinely cares and has not the capacity for risking harm or danger has to define himself, both to himself and to others, as a coward.

I take it then that from the standpoint of those types of relationship without which practices cannot be sustained truthfulness, justice and courage – and perhaps some others – are genuine excellences, are virtues in the light of which we have to characterise ourselves and others, whatever our private moral standpoint or our society's particular codes may be. For this recognition that we cannot escape the definition of our relationships in terms of such goods is perfectly compatible with the acknowledgment that different societies have and have had different codes of truthfulness, justice and courage. Lutheran pietists brought up their children to believe that one ought to tell the truth to everybody at all times, whatever the circumstances or consequences, and Kant was one of their children. Traditional Bantu parents brought up their children not to tell the truth to unknown strangers, since they believed that this could render the family vulnerable to witchcraft. In our culture many of us have been brought up not to tell the truth to elderly great-aunts who invite us to admire their new hats. But each of these codes embodies an acknowledgment of the virtue of truthfulness. So it is also with varying codes of justice and of courage.

Practices then might flourish in societies with very different codes; what they could not do is flourish in societies in which the virtues were not valued, although institutions and technical skills serving unified purposes might well continue to flourish. (I shall have more to say about the contrast between institutions and technical skills mobilised for a unified end, on the one hand, and practices on the other, in a moment.) For the kind of cooperation, the kind of recognition of authority and of achievement, the kind of respect for standards and the kind of risk-taking which are characteristically involved in practices demand for example fairness in judging oneself and others – the kind of fairness absent in my example of the professor – a ruthless truthfulness without which fairness cannot find application – the kind of truthfulness absent in my example of A, B, C and D – and willingness to trust the judgments of those whose achievement in the practice give them an authority to judge which presupposes fairness and truthfulness in those judgments, and from time to time the taking of self-endangering, reputation-endangering and even achievement-endangering risks. It is no part of my thesis that great violinists cannot be vicious or great chess-players mean-spirited. Where the virtues are required, the vices also may flourish. It is just that the vicious and mean-spirited necessarily rely on the virtues of others for the practices in which they engage to flourish and also deny themselves the experience of achieving those internal goods which may reward even not very good chess-players and violinists.

To situate the virtues any further within practices it is necessary now to clarify a little further the nature of a practice by drawing two important contrasts. The discussion so far I hope makes it clear that a practice, in the sense intended, is never just a set of technical skills, even when directed towards some unified purpose and even if the exercise of those skills can on occasion be valued or enjoyed for their own sake. What is distinctive of a practice is in part the way in which conceptions of the relevant goods and ends which the technical skills serve – and every practice does require the exercise of technical skills – are transformed and enriched by these extensions of human powers and by that regard for its own internal goods which are partially definitive of each particular practice or type of practice. Practices never have a goal or goals fixed for all time – painting has no such goal nor has physics – but the goals themselves are transmuted by the history of the activity. It therefore turns out not to be accidental that every practice has its own history and a history which is more and other than that of the improvement of the relevant technical skills. This historical dimension is crucial in relation to the virtues.

To enter into a practice is to enter into a relationship not only with its contemporary practitioners, but also with those who have preceded us in the practice, particularly those whose achievements extended the reach of the practice to its present point. It is thus the achievement, and *a fortiori* the authority, of a tradition which I then confront and from which I have to learn. And for this learning and the relationship to the past which it embodies the virtues of justice, courage and truthfulness are prerequisite in precisely the same way and for precisely the same reasons as they are in sustaining present relationships within practices.

It is not only of course with sets of technical skills that practices ought to be contrasted. Practices must not be confused with institutions. Chess, physics and medicine are practices; chess clubs, laboratories, universities and hospitals are institutions. Institutions are characteristically and necessarily concerned with what I have called external goods. They are involved in acquiring money and other material goods; they are structured in terms of power and status, and they distribute money, power and status as rewards. Nor could they do otherwise if they are to sustain not only themselves, but also the practices of which they are the bearers. For no practices can survive for any length of time unsustained by institutions. Indeed so intimate is the relationship of practices to institutions – and consequently of the goods external to the goods internal to the practices in question – that institutions and practices characteristically form a single causal order in which the ideals and the creativity of the practice are always vulnerable to the acquisitiveness of the institution, in which the cooperative care for common goods of the practice is always vulnerable to the competitiveness of the institution. In this context the essential function of the virtues is clear. Without them, without justice, courage and truthfulness, practices could not resist the corrupting power of institutions.

Yet if institutions do have corrupting power, the making and sustaining of forms of human community – and therefore of institutions – itself has all the characteristics of a practice, and moreover of a practice which stands in a peculiarly close relationship to the exercise of the virtues in two important ways. The exercise of the virtues is itself apt to require a highly determinate attitude to social and political issues; and it is always within some particular community with its own specific institutional forms that we learn or fail to learn to exercise the virtues. There is of course a crucial difference between the way in which the relationship between moral character and political community is envisaged from the standpoint of liberal individualist modernity and the way in which that relationship was envisaged from the standpoint of the type of ancient and medieval tradition of the virtues which I have sketched. For liberal individualism a community is simply an arena in which individuals each pursue their own self-chosen conception of the good life, and political institutions exist to provide that degree of order which makes such self-determined activity possible. Government and law are, or ought to be, neutral between rival conceptions of the good life for man, and hence, although it is the task of government to promote law-abidingness, it is on the liberal view no part of the legitimate function of government to inculcate any one moral outlook.

By contrast, on the particular ancient and medieval view which I have sketched political community not only requires the exercise of the virtues for its own sustenance, but it is one of the tasks of government to make its citizens virtuous, just as it is one of the tasks of parental authority to make children grow up so as to be virtuous adults. The classical statement of this analogy is by Socrates in the *Crito*. It does not of course follow from an acceptance of the Socratic view of political community and political authority that we ought to assign to the modern state the moral function which Socrates assigned to the city and its laws. Indeed the power of the liberal individualist standpoint partly derives from the evident fact that the modern state is indeed totally unfitted to act as moral educator of any community. But the history of how the modern state emerged is of course itself a moral history. If my account of the complex relationship of virtues to practices and to institutions is correct, it follows that we shall be unable to write a true history of practices and institutions unless that history is also one of the virtues and vices. For the ability of a practice to retain its integrity will depend on the way in which the virtues can be and are exercised in sustaining the institutional forms which are the social bearers of the practice. The integrity of a practice causally requires the exercise of the virtues by at least some of the individuals who embody it in their activities; and conversely the corruption of institutions is always in part at least an effect of the vices.

The virtues are of course themselves in turn fostered by certain types of social institution and endangered by others. Thomas Jefferson thought that only in a society of small farmers could the virtues flourish; and Adam Ferguson with a good deal more sophistication saw the institutions of modern commercial society as endangering at least some traditional virtues. It is Ferguson's type of sociology which is the empirical counterpart of the conceptual account of the virtues which I have given, a sociology which aspires to lay bare the empirical, causal connection between virtues, practices and institutions. For this kind of conceptual account has strong empirical implications; it provides an explanatory scheme which can be tested in particular cases. Moreover my thesis has empirical content in another way; it does entail that without the virtues there could be a recognition only of what I have called external goods and not at all of internal goods in the context of practices. And in any society which recognised only external goods competitiveness would be the dominant and even exclusive feature. We have a brilliant portrait of such a society in Hobbes's account of the state of nature; and Professor Turnbull's report of the fate of the Ik suggests that social reality does in the most horrifying way confirm both my thesis and Hobbes's.

Virtues then stand in a different relationship to external and to internal goods. The possession of the virtues – and not only of their semblance and simulacra – is necessary to achieve the latter; yet the possession of the virtues may perfectly well hinder us in achieving external goods. I need to emphasise at this point that external goods genuinely are goods. Not only are they characteristic objects of human desire, whose allocation is what gives point to the virtues of justice and of generosity, but no one can despise them altogether without a certain hypocrisy. Yet notoriously the cultivation of truthfulness, justice and courage will often, the world being what it contingently is, bar us from being rich or famous or powerful. Thus although we may hope that we can not only achieve the standards of excellence and the internal goods of certain practices by possessing the virtues *and* become rich, famous and powerful, the virtues are always a potential stumbling block to this comfortable ambition. We should therefore expect that, if in a particular society the pursuit of external goods were to become dominant, the concept of the virtues might suffer first attrition and then perhaps something near total effacement, although simulacra might abound.

The time has come to ask the question of how far this partial account of a core conception of the virtues – and I need to emphasise that all that I have offered so far is the first stage of such an account – is faithful to the tradition which I delineated. How far, for example, and in what ways is it Aristotelian? It is – happily – not Aristotelian in two ways in which a good deal of the rest of the tradition also dissents from Aristotle. First, although this account of the virtues is teleological, it does not require the identification of any teleology in nature, and hence it does not require any allegiance to Aristotle's metaphysical biology. And secondly, just because of the multiplicity of human practices and the consequent multiplicity of goods in the pursuit of which the virtues may be exercised – goods which will often be contingently incompatible and which will therefore make rival claims upon our allegiance – conflict will not spring solely from flaws in individual character. But it was just on these two matters that Aristotle's account of the virtues seemed most vulnerable; hence if it turns out to be the case that this socially teleological account can support Aristotle's general account of the virtues as well as does his own biologically teleological account, these differences from Aristotle himself may well be regarded as strengthening rather than weakening the case for a generally Aristotelian standpoint.

There are at least three ways in which the account that I have given *is* clearly Aristotelian. First it requires for its completion a cogent elaboration of just those distinctions and concepts which Aristotle's account requires:

voluntariness, the distinction between the intellectual virtues and the virtues of character, the relationship of both to natural abilities and to the passions and the structure of practical reasoning. On every one of these topics something very like Aristotle's view has to be defended, if my own account is to be plausible.

Secondly my account can accommodate an Aristotelian view of pleasure and enjoyment, whereas it is interestingly irreconcilable with any utilitarian view and more particularly with Franklin's account of the virtues. We can approach these questions by considering how to reply to someone who, having considered my account of the differences between goods internal to and goods external to a practice enquired into which class, if either, does pleasure or enjoyment fall? The answer is, 'Some types of pleasure into one, some into the other.'

Someone who achieves excellence in a practice, who plays chess or football well or who carries through an enquiry in physics or an experimental mode in painting with success, characteristically enjoys his achievement and his activity in achieving. So does someone who, although not breaking the limit of achievement, plays or thinks or acts in a way that leads towards such a breaking of limit. As Aristotle says, the enjoyment of the activity and the enjoyment of achievement are not the ends at which the agent aims, but the enjoyment supervenes upon the successful activity in such a way that the activity achieved and the activity enjoyed are one and the same state. Hence to aim at the one is to aim at the other; and hence also it is easy to confuse the pursuit of excellence with the pursuit of enjoyment *in this specific sense*. This particular confusion is harmless enough; what is not harmless is the confusion of enjoyment *in this specific sense* with other forms of pleasure.

For certain kinds of pleasure are of course external goods along with prestige, status, power and money. Not all pleasure is the enjoyment supervening upon achieved activity; some is the pleasure of psychological or physical states independent of all activity. Such states – for example that produced on a normal palate by the closely successive and thereby blended sensations of Colchester oyster, cayenne pepper and Veuve Cliquot – may be sought as external goods, as external rewards which may be purchased by money or received in virtue of prestige. Hence the pleasures are categorised neatly and appropriately by the classification into internal and external goods.

It is just this classification which can find no place within Franklin's account of the virtues which is formed entirely in terms of external relationships and external goods. Thus although by this stage of the argument it is possible to claim that my account does capture a conception of the virtues which is at the core of the particular ancient and medieval tradition which I have delineated, it is equally clear that there is more than one possible conception of the virtues and that Franklin's standpoint and indeed any utilitarian standpoint is such that to accept it will entail rejecting the tradition and *vice versa*.

One crucial point of incompatibility was noted long ago by D. H. Lawrence. When Franklin asserts, 'Rarely use venery but for health or offspring . . .', Lawrence replies, 'Never *use* venery.' It is of the character of a virtue that in order that it be effective in producing the internal goods which are the rewards of the virtues it should be exercised without regard to consequences. For it turns out to be the case that – and this is in part at least one more empirical factual claim – although the virtues are just those qualities which tend to lead to the achievement of a certain class of goods, none the less unless we practice them irrespective of whether in any particular set of contingent circumstances they will produce those goods or not, we cannot possess them at all. We cannot be genuinely courageous or truthful and be so only on occasion. Moreover, as we have seen, cultivation of the virtues always may and often does hinder the achievement of those external goods which are the mark of worldly success. The road to success in Philadelphia and the road to heaven may not coincide after all.

Furthermore we are now able to specify one crucial difficulty for *any* version of utilitarianism – in addition to those which I noticed earlier. Utilitarianism cannot accommodate the distinction between goods internal to and goods external to a practice. Not only is that distinction marked by none of the classical utilitarians – it cannot be found in Bentham's writings nor in those of either of the Mills or of Sidgwick – but internal goods and external goods are not commensurable with each other. Hence the notion of summing goods – and *a fortiori* in the light of what I have said about kinds of pleasure and enjoyment the notion of summing happiness – in terms of one single formula or conception of utility, whether it is Franklin's or Bentham's or Mill's, makes no sense. None the less we ought to note that although *this* distinction is alien to J. S. Mill's thought, it is plausible and in no way patronising to suppose that something like this is the distinction which he was trying to make in *Utilitarianism* when he distinguished between 'higher' and 'lower' pleasures. At the most we can say 'something like this'; for J. S. Mill's upbringing had given him a limited view of human life and powers, had unfitted him, for example, for appreciating games just because of the way it had fitted him for appreciating philosophy. None the less the notion that the pursuit of excellence in a way that extends human powers is at the heart of human life is instantly recognisable as at home in not only J. S. Mill's political and social thought, but also in his and Mrs Taylor's life. Were I to choose human exemplars of certain of the virtues as I understand them, there would of course be many names to name, those of St Benedict and St Francis of Assisi and St Theresa *and* those of Frederick Engels and Eleanor Marx and Leon Trotsky among them. But that of John Stuart Mill would have to be there as certainly as any other.

Thirdly my account is Aristotelian in that it links evaluation and explanation in a characteristically Aristotelian way. From an Aristotelian standpoint to identify certain actions as manifesting or failing to manifest a virtue or virtues is never only to evaluate; it is also to take the first step towards explaining why those actions rather than some others were performed. Hence for an Aristotelian quite as much as for a Platonist the fate of a city or an individual can be explained by citing the injustice of a tyrant or the courage of its defenders. Indeed without allusion to the place that justice and injustice, courage and cowardice play in human life very little will be genuinely explicable. It follows that many of the explanatory projects of the modern social sciences, a methodological canon of which is the separation of 'the facts' – this conception of 'the facts' is the one which I delineated in an earlier chapter – from all evaluation, are bound to fail. For the fact that someone was or failed to be courageous or just cannot be recognised as 'a fact' by those who accept that methodological canon. The account of the virtues which I have given is completely at one with Aristotle's on this point. But now the question may be raised: your account may be in many respects Aristotelian, but is it not in some respects false? Consider the following important objection.

I have defined the virtues partly in terms of their place in practices. But surely, it may be suggested, some practices – that is, some coherent human activities which answer to the description of what I have called a practice – are evil. So in discussions by some moral philosophers of this type of account of the virtues it has been suggested that torture and sado-masochistic sexual activities might be examples of practices. But how can a disposition be a virtue if it is the kind of disposition which sustains practices and some practices issue in evil? My answer to this objection falls into two parts.

First I want to allow that there *may* be practices – in the sense in which I understand the concept – which simply *are* evil. I am far from convinced that there are, and I do not in fact believe that either torture or sado-masochistic sexuality answer to the description of a practice which my account of the virtues employs. But I do not want to rest my case on this lack of conviction, especially since it is plain that as a matter of contingent fact many types of practice may on particular occasions be productive of evil. For the range of practices includes the arts, the sciences and certain types of intellectual and athletic game. And it is at once obvious that any of these may under certain conditions be a source of evil: the desire to excel and to win can corrupt, a man may be so engrossed by his painting that he neglects his family, what was initially an honourable resort to war can issue in savage cruelty. But what follows from this?

It certainly is not the case that my account entails *either* that we ought to excuse or condone such evils *or* that whatever flows from a virtue is right. I do have to allow that courage sometimes sustains injustice, that loyalty has been known to strengthen a murderous aggressor and that generosity has sometimes weakened the capacity to do good. But to deny this would be to fly in the face of just those empirical facts which I invoked in criticising Aquinas' account of the unity of the virtues. That the virtues need initially to be defined and explained with reference to the notion of a practice thus in no way entails approval of all practices in all circumstances. That the virtues – as the objection itself presupposed – *are* defined not in terms of good and right practices, but of practices, does not entail or imply that practices as actually carried through at particular times and places do not stand in need of moral criticism. And the resources for such criticism are not lacking. There is in the first place no inconsistency in appealing to the requirements of a virtue to criticise a practice. Justice may be initially defined as a disposition which in its particular way is necessary to sustain practices; it does not follow that in pursuing the requirements of a practice violations of justice are not to be condemned. Moreover I already pointed out in an earlier chapter that a morality of virtues requires as its counterpart a conception of moral law. Its requirements too have to be met by practices. But, it may be asked, does not all this imply that more needs to be said about the place of practices in some larger moral context? Does not this at least suggest that there is more to the core concept of a virtue than can be spelled out in terms of practices? I have after all emphasised that the scope of any virtue in human life extends beyond the practices in terms of which it is initially defined. What then is the place of the virtues in the larger arenas of human life?

I stressed earlier that any account of the virtues in terms of practices could only be a partial and first account. What is required to complement it? The most notable difference so far between my account and any account that could be called Aristotelian is that although I have in no way restricted the exercise of the virtues to the context of practices, it is in terms of practices that I have located their point and function. Whereas Aristotle locates that point and function in terms of the notion of a type of whole human life which can be called good. And it does seem that the question 'What would a human being lack who lacked the virtues?' must be given a kind of answer which goes beyond anything which I have said so far. For such an individual would not merely fail *in a variety of particular ways* in respect of the kind of excellence which can be achieved through participation in practices and in respect of the kind of human relationship required to sustain such excellence. His own life *viewed as a whole* would perhaps be defective; it would not be the kind of life which someone would describe in trying to answer the question 'What is the best kind of life for this kind of man or woman to live?' And that question cannot be answered without at least raising Aristotle's own question, 'What is the good life for man?' Consider three ways in which a human life informed only by the conception of the virtues sketched so far would be defective.

It would be pervaded, first of all, by *too many* conflicts and *too much* arbitrariness. I argued earlier that it is a merit of an account of the virtues in terms of a multiplicy of goods that it allows for the possibility of tragic conflict in a way in which Aristotle's does not. But it may also produce even in the life of someone who is virtuous and disciplined too many occasions when one allegiance points in one direction, another in another. The claims of one practice may be incompatible with another in such a way that one may find oneself oscillating in an arbitrary way, rather than making rational choices. So it seems to have been with T. E. Lawrence. Commitment to sustaining the kind of community in which the virtues can flourish may be incompatible with the devotion which a particular practice – of the arts, for example – requires. So there may be tensions between the claims of family life and those of the arts – the problem that Gauguin solved or failed to solve by fleeing to Polynesia, or between the claims of politics and those of the arts – the problem that Lenin solved or failed to solve by refusing to listen to Beethoven.

If the life of the virtues is continuously fractured by choices in which one allegiance entails the apparently arbitrary renunciation of another, it may seem that the goods internal to practices do after all derive their authority from our individual choices; for when different goods summon in different and in incompatible directions, 'I' have to choose between their rival claims. The modern self with its criterionless choices apparently reappears in the alien context of what was claimed to be an Aristotelian world. This accusation might be rebutted in part by returning to the question of why both goods and virtues do have authority in our lives and repeating what was said earlier in this chapter. But this reply would only be partly successful; the distinctively modern notion of choice would indeed have reappeared, even if with a more limited scope for its exercise than it has usually claimed.

Secondly without an overriding conception of the *telos* of a whole human life, conceived as a unity, our conception of certain individual virtues has to remain partial and incomplete. Consider two examples. Justice, on an Aristotelian view, is defined in terms of giving each person his or her due or desert. To deserve well is to have contributed in some substantial way to the achievement of those goods, the sharing of which and the common pursuit of which provide foundations for human community. But the goods internal to practices, including the goods internal to the practice of making and sustaining forms of community, need to be ordered and evaluated in some way if we are to assess relative desert. Thus only substantive application of an Aristotelian concept of justice requires an understanding of goods and of the good that goes beyond the multiplicity of goods which inform practices. As with justice, so also with patience. Patience is the virtue of waiting attentively without complaint, but not of waiting thus for anything at all. To treat patience as a virtue presupposes some adequate answer to the question: waiting for what? Within the context of practices a partial, although for many purposes adequate, answer can be given: the patience of a craftsman with refractory material, of a teacher with a slow pupil, of a politician in negotiations, are all species of patience. But what if the material is just too refractory, the pupil too slow, the negotiations too frustrating? Ought we always at a certain point just to give up in the interests of the practice itself? The medieval exponents of the virtue of patience claimed that there are certain types of situation in which the virtue of patience requires that I do not ever give up on some person or task, situations in which, as they would have put it, I am required to embody in my attitude to that person or task something of the patient attitude of God towards his creation. But this could only be so if patience served some overriding good, some *telos* which warranted putting other goods in a subordinate place. Thus it turns out that the content of the virtue of patience depends upon how we order various goods in a hierarchy and *a fortiori* on whether we are able rationally so to order these particular goods.

I have suggested so far that unless there is a *telos* which transcends the limited goods of practices by constituting the good of a whole human life, the good of a human life conceived as a unity, it will *both* be the case that a certain subversive arbitrariness will invade the moral life *and* that we shall be unable to specify the context of certain virtues adequately. These two considerations are reinforced by a third: that there is at least one virtue recognised by the tradition which cannot be specified at all except with reference to the wholeness of a human life – the virtue of integrity or constancy. 'Purity of heart,' said Kierkegaard, 'is to will one thing.' This notion of singleness of purpose in a whole life can have no application unless that of a whole life does.

It is clear therefore that my preliminary account of the virtues in terms of practices captures much, but very far from all, of what the Aristotelian tradition taught about the virtues. It is also clear that to give an account that is at once more fully adequate to the tradition and rationally defensible, it is necessary to raise a question to which the Aristotelian tradition presupposed an answer, an answer so widely shared in the pre-modern world that it never had to be formulated explicitly in any detailed way. This question is: is it rationally justifiable to conceive of each human life as a unity, so that we may try to specify each such life as having its good and so that we may understand the virtues as having their function in enabling an individual to make of his or her life one kind of unity rather than another?

7

What Do Women Want in a Moral Theory?

Annette Baier

When I finished reading Carol Gilligan's *In a Different Voice*,[1] I asked myself the obvious question for a philosopher reader: what differences should one expect in the moral philosophy done by women, supposing Gilligan's sample of women to be representative and supposing her analysis of their moral attitudes and moral development to be correct? Should one expect women to want to produce moral theories, and if so, what sort of moral theories? How will any moral theories they produce differ from those produced by men?

Obviously one does not have to make this an entirely a priori and hypothetical question. One can look and see what sort of contributions women have made to moral philosophy. Such a look confirms, I think, Gilligan's findings. What one finds *is* a bit different in tone and approach from the standard sort of moral philosophy as done by men following in the footsteps of the great moral philosophers (all men). Generalizations are extremely rash, but when I think of Philippa Foot's work on the moral virtues, Elizabeth Anscombe's work on intention and on modern moral philosophy, Iris Murdoch's philosophical writings, Ruth Barcan Marcus's work on moral dilemmas, the work of the radical feminist moral philosophers who are not content with orthodox Marxist lines of thought, Jenny Teichman's book on illegitimacy, Susan Wolf's articles, Claudia Card's essay on mercy, Sabina Lovibond's writings, Gabriele Taylor's work on pride, love, and on integrity, Cora Diamond's and Mary Midgeley's work on our attitude toward animals, Sissela Bok's work on lying and on secrecy, Virginia Held's work, the work of Alison Jaggar, Marilyn Frye, and many others, I seem to hear a different voice from the

Annette Baier, "What Do Women Want in a Moral Theory?" *Moral Prejudices* (Cambridge, MA: Harvard University Press, 1994), pp. 1–17.

standard moral philosophers' voice. I hear the voice Gilligan heard, made reflective and philosophical. What women want in moral philosophy is what they are providing. And what they are providing seems to me to confirm Gilligan's theses about women. One has to be careful here, of course, for not all important contributions to moral philosophy by women fall easily into the Gilligan stereotype or its philosophical extension. Nor has it been only women who have been proclaiming discontent with the standard approach in moral philosophy and trying new approaches. Michael Stocker, Alasdair MacIntyre, and Ian Hacking when he assesses the game-theoretic approach to morality,[2] all should be given the status of honorary women, if we accept the hypothesis that there are some moral insights for whatever reason women seem to attain more easily or more reliably than men do. Still, exceptions confirm the rule, so I shall proceed undaunted by these important exceptions to my generalizations.

If Hacking is right, preoccupation with prisoner's and prisoners' dilemmas is a big boys' game, and a pretty silly one too. It is, I think, significant that women have not rushed into the field of game-theoretic moral philosophy, and that those who have dared enter that male locker room have said distinctive things there. Edna Ullmann Margalit's book *The Emergence of Norms* put prisoner's dilemma in its limited moral place. Supposing that at least part of the explanation for the relatively few women in this field is disinclination rather than disability, one might ask if this disinclination also extends to the construction of moral theories. For although we find out what sort of moral philosophy women want by looking to see what they have provided, if we do that for moral theory, the answer we get seems to be "none." None of the contributions to moral philosophy by women really counts as a moral theory, nor is seen as such by its author.

Is it that reflective women, when they become philosophers, want to do without moral theory, want no part in the construction of such theories? To conclude this at this early stage, when we have only a few generations of women moral philosophers to judge from, would be rash indeed. The term "theory" can be used in wider and narrower ways, and in its widest sense a moral theory is simply an internally consistent fairly comprehensive account of what morality is and when and why it merits our acceptance and support. In that wide sense, a moral theory is something it would take a skeptic, or one who believes that our intellectual vision is necessarily blurred or distorted when we let it try to take in too much, to be an antitheorist. Even if there were some truth in the latter claim, one might compatibly with it still hope to build up a coherent total account by a mosaic method, assembling a lot of smaller-scale works until one had built up a complete account – say, taking the virtues or purported virtues one by one until one had a more or less complete account. But would that sort of comprehensiveness in one's moral philosophy entitle one to call the finished work a moral theory? If it would, then many women moral philosophers today can be seen as engaged in moral theory construction. In the weakest sense of "theory," as a coherent near-comprehensive account, there are plenty of incomplete theories to be found in the works of women moral philosophers. And in *that* sense of theory, most of what are recognized as the current moral theories are also incomplete, because they do not yet purport to be really comprehensive. Wrongs to animals and wrongful destruction of our physical environment are put to one side by John Rawls, and in most "liberal" theories there are only hand waves concerning our proper attitude toward our children, toward the ill, toward our relatives, friends, and lovers.

Is comprehensiveness too much to ask of a moral theory? The paradigm examples of moral theories – those that are called by their authors "moral theories" – are distinguished not by the comprehensiveness of their internally coherent account but by the *sort* of coherence which is aimed at over a fairly broad area. Their method is not the mosaic method but the broad brushstroke method. Moral theories, as we know them, are, to change the art form, vaults rather than walls – they are not built by assembling painstakingly made brick after brick. In *this* sense of theory – a fairly tightly systematic account of a large area of morality, with a keystone supporting all the rest – women moral philosophers have not yet, to my knowledge, produced moral theories or claimed that they have.

Leaving to one side the question of what purpose (other than good clean intellectual fun) is served by such moral theories, and supposing for the sake of argument that women can, if they wish, systematize as well as the next man and, if need be, systematize in a mathematical fashion as well as the next mathematically minded moral philosopher, then what key concept or guiding motif might hold together the structure of a moral theory hypothetically produced by a reflective woman, Gilligan-style, who has taken up moral theorizing as a calling? What would be a suitable central question, principle, or concept to structure a moral theory which might accommodate those moral insights which women tend to have more readily than men, and to answer those moral questions which, it seems, worry women more than men? I hypothesized that the women's theory, expressive mainly of women's insights and concerns, would be an ethics of love, and this hypothesis seems to be Gilligan's too, since she has gone on from *In a Different Voice* to write about the limitations of Freud's understanding of love as women know it.[3] But presumably women theorists will be like enough to men to want their moral theory to be acceptable to all, so acceptable both to reflective women and to reflective men. Like any good theory, it will need not to ignore the partial truth of previous theories. It must therefore accommodate both the insights men have more easily than women and those women have more easily than men. It should swallow up its predecessor theories. Women moral theorists, if any, will have this very great advantage over the men whose theories theirs supplant, that they can stand on the shoulders of male moral theorists, as no man has yet been able to stand on the shoulders of any female moral theorist. There can be advantages as well as handicaps in being latecomers. So women theorists will need to connect their ethics of love with what has been the men theorists' preoccupation, namely, obligation.

The great and influential moral theorists have in the modern era taken *obligation* as the key and the problematic concept, and have asked what justifies treating a person as morally bound or obliged to do a particular thing. Since to be bound is to be unfree, by making obligation central one at the same time makes central the question of the justification of coercion, of forcing or trying to force someone to act in a particular way. The concept of obligation as justified limitation of freedom does just what one wants a good theoretical concept to do – to divide up the field (as one looks at different ways one's freedom may be limited, freedom in different spheres, different sorts and versions and levels of justification) and at the same time to hold the subfields together. There must in a theory be some generalization and some speciation or diversification, and a good rich key concept guides one both in recognizing the diversity and in recognizing the unity in it. The concept of obligation has served this function very well for the area of morality it covers, and so we have some fine theories about that area. But as Aristotelians and Christians, as well as women, know, there is a lot of morality *not* covered by that concept, a lot of very great importance even for the area where there are obligations.

This is fairly easy to see if we look at what lies behind the perceived obligation to keep promises. Unless there is some good moral reason why someone should assume the responsibility of rearing a child to be *capable* of taking promises seriously, once she understands what a promise is, the obligation to obey promises will not effectively tie her, and any force applied to punish her when she breaks promises or makes fraudulent ones will be of questionable justice. Is there an *obligation* on someone to make the child into a morally competent promisor? If so, on whom? Who has failed in his or her obligations when, say, war orphans who grew up without parental love or any other love arrive at legal adulthood very willing to be untrue to their word? Who failed in what obligation in all those less extreme cases of attempted but unsuccessful moral education? The parents who didn't produce promise-keeping offspring? Those who failed to educate the parents in how to educate their children (whoever it might be who could plausibly be thought to have the responsibility for training parents to fulfill their obligations)? The liberal version of our basic moral obligations tends to be fairly silent on who has what obligations to new members of the moral community, and it would throw most theories of the justification of obligations into some confusion if the obligation to rear one's children lovingly were added to the list of obligations. Such evidence as we have about the conditions in which children do successfully "learn" the morality of the community of which they are members suggests that we cannot substitute "conscientiously" for "lovingly" in this hypothetical extra needed obligation. But an obligation to love, in the strong sense needed, would be an embarrassment to the theorist, given most accepted versions of "ought implies can."

It is hard to make fair generalizations here, so I shall content myself with indicating how this charge I am making against the current men's moral theories, that their version of the justified list of obligations does not ensure the proper care of the young and so does nothing to ensure the stability of the morality in question over several generations, can be made against what I regard as the best of the men's recent theories, Rawls's theory of justice. One of the great strengths of Rawls's theory is the careful attention given to the question of how just institutions produce the conditions for their continued support, across generations, and in particular of how the sense of justice will arise in children, once there are minimally just institutions structuring the social world into which they are born. Rawls, more than most moral theorists, has attended to the question of the stability of his just society, given what we know about child development. But Rawls's sensitive account of the conditions for the development of that sense of justice needed for the maintenance of his version of a just society takes it for granted that there will be loving parents rearing the children in whom the sense of justice is to develop. "The parents, we may suppose, love the child, and in time the child comes to love and trust the parents." Why may we suppose this? Not because compliance with Rawls's version of our obligations and duties will ensure it. Rawls's theory, like so many other theories of obligation, in the end must take out a loan not only on the natural duty of parents to care for children (which he will have no trouble including) but on the natural *virtue* of parental love (or even a loan on the maternal instinct?). The virtue of being a *loving* parent must supplement the natural duties and the obligations of justice, if the just society is to last beyond the first generation. And as Nancy Chodorow's work indicates, the loving parents must also accept a certain division of child-care responsibility if their version of the obligations and virtues of men and of women is, along with their version of the division of labor accompanying that allocation of virtues, to be passed on.

Reliance on a recognized obligation to turn oneself into a good parent or else to avoid becoming a parent would be a problematic solution. Good parents tend to be the children of good parents, so this obligation would collapse into the obligation to avoid parenthood unless one expected to be a good parent. That, given available methods of contraception, may itself convert into the obligation, should one expect not to be a good parent, to sexual abstinence, or sterilization, or resolute resort to abortion when contraception fails. The conditional obligation to abort, and in effect also the conditional obligation to sterilization, falls on the women. There may be conditions in which the rational moral choice is between obligatory sexual abstinence and obligatory sterilization, but obligatory abortion, such as women in China now face, seems to me a moral monster. I do not believe that liberal moral theorists will be able to persuade reflective women that a morality that in any conditions makes abortion obligatory, as distinct from permitted or advisable or, on occasion, best, is in their own as well as their male fellows' long-term self-interest. It would be tragic if such moral questions in the end came to the question of whose best interests to sacrifice, men's or women's. I do not believe they *do* come to this, but should they, then justice would require that, given the long history of the subordination of women's to men's interests, men's interests be sacrificed. Justice, of course, never decides these issues unless power reinforces justice, so I am not predicting any victory for women, should it ever come to a fight over obligatory abortion or over who is to face obligatory sterilization.

No liberal moral theorist, as far as I know, is advocating obligatory abortion or obligatory sterilization when necessary to prevent the conception of children whose parents do not expect to love them. My point rather is that they escape this conclusion only by avoiding the issue of what is to ensure that new members of the moral community do get the loving care they need to become morally competent persons. Liberal moral theories assume that women either will provide loving maternal care, or will persuade their mates to provide loving paternal care, or when pregnant will decide for abortion, encouraged by their freedom-loving men. These theories, in other words, exploit the culturally encouraged maternal instinct and/or the culturally encouraged docility of women. The liberal system would receive a nasty spanner in its works should women use their freedom of choice as regards abortion to choose *not* to abort, and then leave their newborn children on their fathers' doorsteps. That would test liberal morality's ability to provide for its own survival.

At this point it may be objected that every moral theory must make some assumptions about the natural psychology of those on whom obligations are imposed. Why shouldn't the liberal theory count on a continuing sufficient supply of good loving mothers, as it counts on continuing self-interest and, perhaps, on a continuing supply of pugnacious men who are able and willing to become good soldiers, without turning any of these into moral *obligations*? Why waste moral resources recognizing as obligatory or as virtuous what one can count on getting without moral pressure? If, in the moral economy, one can get enough good mothers and good warriors "for free," why not gladly exploit what nature and cultural history offer? I cannot answer this question fully here, but my argument does depend upon the assumption that a decent morality will *not* depend for its stability on forces to which it gives no moral recognition. Its account books should be open to scrutiny, and there should be no unpaid debts, no loans with no prospect of repayment. I also assume that once we are clear about these matters and about the interdependencies involved, out principles of justice will not allow us to recognize either a special obligation on every woman to initiate the killing of the fetus she has conceived, should she and her mate be, or think they will be, deficient in parental love, or a special obligation on every young man to kill those his elders have labeled enemies of his country. Both such "obligations" are prima facie suspect, and difficult to make consistent with any of the principles supposedly generating obligations in modern moral theories. I also assume that, on reflection, we will not want to recognize as *virtues* the character traits of women and men which lead them to supply such life and death services "for free." Neither maternal servitude, nor the resoluteness needed to kill off one's children to prevent their growing up unloved, nor the easy willingness to go out and kill when ordered to do so by authorities seems to me to be a character trait a decent morality will encourage by labeling it a virtue. But the liberals' morality must somehow encourage such traits if its stability depends on enough people showing them. There is, then, understandable motive for liberals' avoidance of the question of whether such qualities are or are not morally approved of, and of whether or not there is any obligation to act as one with such character traits would act.

It is symptomatic of the bad faith of liberal morality as understood by many of those who defend it that issues such as whether to fight or not to fight, to have or not to have an abortion, or to be or not to be an unpaid maternal drudge are left to individual conscience. Since there is no coherent guidance liberal morality can give on these issues, which clearly are *not* matters of moral indifference, liberal morality tells each of us, "the choice is yours," hoping that enough will choose to be self-sacrificial life providers and self-sacrificial death dealers to suit the purposes of the rest.

Rawls's theory does explicitly face the question of the moral justification of refusal to bear arms, and of how a just society justly provides for its own defense. The hardships imposed on conscripted soldiers are, he says, a necessary evil, and the most that just institutions can do is to "make sure that the risks of suffering from those misfortunes are more or less evenly shared by all members of society over the course of their life, and that there is no avoidable class bias in selecting those who are called for duty." What of sex/gender bias? Or is that assumed to be unavoidable? Rawls's principles seem to me to imply that women should be conscripted, if anyone is (and I think that is right), but since he avoids the questions of justice between men and women one does not know whether he intended this implication. His suggestion that one argument in favor of a conscripted army is that it is less likely to be an instrument of unjustified foreign adventures will become even stronger, I believe, if half the conscripts are women. Like most male moral theorists, Rawls does not discuss the morality of having children, refusing to have them, refusing to care for them, nor does he discuss how just institutions might equalize the responsibilities involved in ensuring that there be new members of society and that they become morally competent members of it, so one does not know whether he accepts a gender-based division of social service here, leaving it to the men to do the dangerous defensive destruction of life and cities, while the support of new life, and any costs going or contrived to go with that, are left to the women. I hope that is not what he meant.

I do not wish, by having myself spoken of these two traditionally gender-based allocations of responsibility (producing and caring for new human life and the destruction of the lives of those officially labeled enemies) together, to leave the impression that I see any parallel between them except that they have both been treated as gender based and that both present embarrassments for liberal moral theory. Not all allocations of responsibility are allocations of burdens, and parenthood, unlike unchosen military life, need not be seen as essentially burden bearing. Good mothers and good soldiers make contributions of very different sorts and sort of importance to the ongoing life of a moral community, and they should not be seen, as they sometimes are, as fair mutual substitutes, as forms of social service. Good mothers will always be needed by a moral community, in the best conditions as well as the worst; the need for good military men, though foreseeably permanent, is a sign of some failure of our morality, a failure of our effectively acted upon moral laws to be valid theorems for the conservation of men in multitudes. Nor do the burdens of soldiering have any real analogue in the case of motherhood, which today *need* not impose real costs on the mother. If there are significant costs – loss of career opportunity, improperly recompensed drudgery in the home, or health risks – this is due to bad but largely remediable social arrangements, as the failure of parents to experience any especially parental satisfactions may be also due to bad but remediable socially produced attitudes toward parental responsibility. We do not, I think, want our military men to enjoy killing the enemy and destroying their cities, and any changes we made in social customs and institutions to make such pleasures more likely would be deplorable ones. Military life in wartime should always be seen as a sacrifice, while motherhood should never need to be seen as self-sacrificial service. If it is an honor and a privilege to bear arms for one's country, as we understandably tell our military conscripts and volunteers, part of the honor is being trusted with activities that are a necessary evil, being trusted not to enjoy their evil aspects, and being trusted to see the evil as well as the necessity. Only if we contrive to make the bringing into the world of new persons as nasty a business as killing already present persons will there be any just reason to exclude young women from conscripted armies or to exclude men from equal parental responsibility.

Granted that the men's theories of obligation need supplementation, to have much chance of integrity and coherence, and that the women's hypothetical theories will want to cover obligation as well as love, then what concept brings them together? My tentative answer is – the concept of appropriate trust, oddly neglected in moral theory. This concept also nicely mediates between reason and feeling, those tired old candidates for moral authority, since to trust is neither quite to believe something about the trusted nor necessarily to feel any emotion toward them – but to have a belief-informed and action-influencing attitude. To make it plausible that the neglected concept of appropriate trust is a good one for the enlightened moral theorist to make central, I need to show, or begin to show, how it could include obligation, indeed shed light on obligations and their justification, as well as include love, the other moral concerns of Gilligan's women, and many of the topics women moral philosophers have chosen to address, mosaic fashion. I would also need to show that it could connect all of these in a way which holds out promise both of synthesis and of comprehensive moral coverage. A moral theory which looked at the conditions for proper trust of all the various sorts we show, and at what sorts of reasons justify inviting such trust, giving it, and meeting it, would, I believe, not have to avoid turning its gaze on the conditions for the survival of the practices it endorses, so it could avoid that unpleasant choice many current liberal theories seem to have – between incoherence and bad faith. I do not pretend that we will easily agree once we raise the questions I think we should raise, but at least we may have a language adequate to the expression of both men's and women's moral viewpoints.

My trust in the concept of trust is based in part on my own attempts to restate and consider what is right and what wrong with men's theories, especially Hume's, which I consider the best of the lot. I have found myself reconstructing his account of the artifices of justice as an account of the progressive enlargement of a climate of trust, and have found that a helpful way to see it. It has some textual basis, but is nevertheless a reconstruction, and one I have found, immodestly, an improvement. So it is because I have tried the concept and explored its dimensions a bit – the variety of goods we may trust others not to take from us, the sort of security or insurance we have when we do, the sorts of defenses or potential defenses we lay down when we trust, the various conditions for reasonable trust of various types – that I am hopeful about its power as a theoretical, and not just an exegetical, tool. I also found myself needing to use it when I made a brief rash attempt at that women's topic, caring (invited in by a male philosopher,[4] I should say). I am reasonably sure that trust does generalize some central moral features of the recognition of binding obligations and moral virtues and of loving, as well as of other important relations between persons, such as teacher–pupil, confider–confidante, worker to co-worker in the same cause, and professional to client. Indeed it is fairly obvious that love, the main moral phenomenon women want attended to, involves trust, so I anticipate little quarrel when I claim that, if we had a moral theory spelling out the conditions for appropriate trust and distrust, that would include a morality of love in all its variants – parental love, love of children for their parents, love of family members, love of friends, of lovers in the strict sense, of co-workers, of one's country and its figureheads, of exemplary heroines and heroes, of goddesses and gods.

Love and loyalty demand maximal trust of one sort, and maximal trustworthiness, and in investigating the conditions for maximal trust and maximal risk we must think about the ethics of love. More controversial may be my claim that the ethics of obligation will also be covered. I see it as covered because to recognize a set of obligations is to trust some group of persons to instill them, to demand that they be met, possibly to levy sanctions if they are not, and this is to trust persons with very significant coercive power over others. Less coercive but still significant power is possessed by those shaping our conception of the virtues and expecting us to display them, approving when we do, disapproving and perhaps shunning us when we do not. Such coercive and manipulative power over others requires justification, and is justified only if we have reason to trust those who have it to use it properly and to use the discretion which is always given when trust is given in a way which serves the purpose of the whole system of moral control, and not merely self-serving or morally improper purposes. Since the question of the justification of coercion becomes, at least in part, the question of the wisdom of trusting the coercers to do their job properly, the morality of obligation, in as far as it reduces to the morality of coercion, is covered by the morality of proper trust. Other forms of trust may also be involved, but trusting enforcers with the use of force is the most problematic form of trust involved.

The coercers and manipulators are, to some extent, all of us, so to ask what our obligations are and what virtues we should exhibit is to ask what it is reasonable to trust us to demand, expect, and contrive to get from one another. It becomes, in part, a question of what powers we can in reason trust ourselves to exercise properly. But self-trust is a dubious or limit case of trust, so I prefer to postpone the examination of the concept of proper self-trust at least until proper trust of others is more clearly understood. Nor do we distort matters too much if we concentrate on those cases where moral sanctions and moral pressure and moral manipulation is not self-applied but applied to others, particularly by older persons to younger persons. Most moral pressuring that has any effect goes on in childhood and early youth. Moral sanctions may continue to be applied, formally and informally, to adults, but unless the criminal courts apply them it is easy enough for adults to ignore them, to brush them aside. It is not difficult to become a sensible knave, and to harden one's heart so that one is insensible to the moral condemnation of one's victims and those who sympathize with them. Only if the pressures applied in the morally formative stage have given one a heart that rebels against the thought of such ruthless independence of what others think will one see any reason *not* to ignore moral condemnation, not to treat it as mere powerless words and breath. Condemning sensible knaves is as much a waste of breath as arguing with them – all we can sensibly do is to try to protect children against their influence, and ourselves against their knavery. Adding to the criminal law will not be the way to do the latter, since such moves will merely challenge sensible knaves to find new knavish exceptions and loopholes, not protect us from sensible knavery. Sensible knaves are precisely those who exploit us without breaking the law. So the whole question of when moral pressure of various sorts, formative, reformative, and punitive, ought to be brought to bear by whom is subsumed under the question of whom to trust when and with what, and for what good reasons.

In concentrating on obligations, rather than virtues, modern moral theorists have chosen to look at the cases where more trust is placed in enforcers of obligations than is placed in ordinary moral agents, the bearers of the obligations. In taking, as contractarians do, contractual obligations as the model of obligations, they concentrate on a case where the very minimal trust is put in the obligated person, and considerable punitive power entrusted to the one to whom the obligation is owed (I assume here that Hume is right in saying that when we promise or contract, we formally subject ourselves to the penalty, in case of failure, of never being trusted as a promisor again). This is an interesting case of the allocation of trust of various sorts, but it surely distorts our moral vision to suppose that *all* obligations, let alone all morally pressured expectations we impose on others, conform to that abnormally coercive model. It takes very special conditions for it to be safe to trust persons to inflict penalties on other persons, conditions in which either we can trust the penalizers to have the virtues necessary to penalize wisely and fairly, or else we can rely on effective threats to keep unvirtuous penalizers from abusing their power – that is to say, rely on others to coerce the first coercers into proper behavior. But that reliance too will either be trust or will have to rely on threats from coercers of the coercers of coercers, and so on. Morality on this model becomes a nasty, if intellectually intriguing, game of mutual mutually corrective threats. The central question of who should deprive whom of what freedom soon becomes the question of whose anger should be dreaded by whom (the theory of obligation), supplemented perhaps by an afterthought on whose favor should be courted by whom (the theory of the virtues).

Undoubtedly some important part of morality does depend in part on a system of threats and bribes, at least for its survival in difficult conditions when normal goodwill and normally virtuous dispositions may be insufficient to motivate the conduct required for the preservation and justice of the moral network of relationships. But equally undoubtedly life will be nasty, emotionally poor, and worse than brutish (even if longer), if that is all morality is, or even if that coercive structure of morality is regarded as the backbone, rather than as an available crutch, should the main support fail. For the main support has to come from those we entrust with the job of rearing and training persons so that they can be trusted in various ways, some trusted with extraordinary coercive powers, some with public decision-making powers, all trusted as parties to promise, most trusted by some who love them and by one or more willing to become co-parents with them, most trusted by dependent children, dependent elderly relatives, sick friends, and so on. A very complex network of a great variety of sorts of trust structures our moral relationships with our fellows, and if there is a *main* support to this network it is the trust we place in those who respond to the trust of new members of the moral community, namely, children, and prepare them for new forms of trust.

A theory which took as its central question "Who should trust whom with what, and why?" would not have to forgo the intellectual fun and games previous theorists have had with the various paradoxes of morality – curbing freedom to increase freedom, curbing self-interest the better to satisfy self-interest, not aiming at happiness in order to become happier. For it is easy enough to get a paradox of trust to accompany or, if I am right, to generalize the paradoxes of freedom, self-interest, and hedonism. To trust is to make oneself or to let oneself be more vulnerable than one might have been to harm from others – to give them an opportunity to harm one, in the confidence that they will not take it, because they have no good reason to. Why would one take such a risk? For risk it always is, given the partial opaqueness to us of the reasoning and motivation of those we trust and with whom we cooperate. Our confidence may be, and quite often is, misplaced. That is what we risk when we trust. If the best reason to take such a risk is the expected gain in security which comes from a climate of trust, then in trusting we are always giving up security to get greater security, exposing our throats so that others become accustomed to not biting. A moral theory which made proper trust its central concern could have its own categorical imperative, could replace obedience to self-made laws and freely chosen restraint on freedom with security-increasing sacrifice of security, distrust in the promoters of a climate of distrust, and so on.

Such reflexive use of one's central concept, negative or affirmative, is an intellectually satisfying activity which is bound to have appeal to those system lovers who want to construct moral theories, and it may help them design their theory in an intellectually pleasing manner. But we should beware of becoming hypnotized by our slogans or of sacrificing truth to intellectual elegance. Any theory of proper trust should not *prejudge* the question of when distrust is proper. We might find more objects of proper distrust than just the contributors to a climate of reasonable distrust, just as freedom should be restricted not just to increase human freedom but to protect human life from poisoners and other killers. I suspect, however, that all the objects of reasonable distrust are more reasonably seen as falling into the category of ones who contribute to a decrease in the scope of proper trust than can all who are reasonably coerced be seen as themselves guilty of wrongful coercion. Still, even if all proper trust turns out to be for such persons and on such matters as will increase the scope or stability of a climate of reasonable trust, and all proper distrust for such persons and on such matters as increase the scope of reasonable distrust, overreliance on such nice reflexive formulae can distract us from asking all the questions about trust which need to be asked if an adequate moral theory is to be constructed around that concept. These questions should include when to *respond* to trust with *un*trustworthiness, when and when not to invite trust, as well as when to give and refuse trust. We should not assume that promiscuous trustworthiness is any more a virtue than is undiscriminating distrust. It is appropriate trustworthiness, appropriate trustingness, appropriate encouragement to trust which will be virtues, as will be judicious untrustworthiness, selective refusal to trust, discriminating discouragement of trust.

Women are particularly well placed to appreciate these last virtues, since they have sometimes needed them to get into a position even to consider becoming moral theorizers. The long exploitation and domination of women by men depended on men's trust in women and women's trustworthiness to play their allotted role and so to perpetuate their own and their daughters' servitude. However keen women now are to end the lovelessness of modern moral philosophy, they are unlikely to lose sight of the cautious virtue of appropriate distrust or of the tough virtue of principled betrayal of the exploiters' trust.

Gilligan's girls and women saw morality as a matter of preserving valued ties to others, of preserving the conditions for that care and mutual care without which human life becomes bleak, lonely, and after a while, as the mature men in her study found, not self-affirming, however successful in achieving the egoistic goals which had been set. The boys and men saw morality as a matter of finding workable traffic rules for self-assertors, so that they not needlessly frustrate one another and so that they could, should they so choose, cooperate in more positive ways to mutual advantage. Both for the women's sometimes unchosen and valued ties with others and for the men's mutual respect as sovereigns and subjects of the same minimal moral traffic rules (and for their more voluntary and more selective associations of profiteers), trust is important. Both men and women are concerned with cooperation, and the dimensions of trust–distrust structure the different cooperative relations each emphasize. The various considerations which arise when we try to defend an answer to any question about the appropriateness of a particular form of cooperation with its distinctive form of trust or distrust, that is, when we look into the terms of all sorts of cooperation, at the terms of trust in different cases of trust, at what are fair terms and what are trust-enhancing and trust-preserving terms, are suitably many and richly interconnected. A moral theory (or family of theories) that made trust its central problem could do better justice to men's and women's moral intuitions than do the going men's theories. Even if we don't easily agree on the answer to the question of who should trust whom with what, who should accept and who should meet various sorts of trust, and why, these questions might enable us better to reason morally together than we can when the central moral questions are reduced to those of whose favor one must court and whose anger one must dread. But such programmatic claims as I am making will be tested only when women standing on the shoulders of men, or men on the shoulders of women, or some theorizing Tiresias actually works out such a theory. I am no Tiresias, and have not foresuffered all the labor pains of such a theory. I aim here only to fertilize.

Postscript

This essay was written before Carol Gilligan had withdrawn the suggestion in *A Different Voice* that there is some intrinsic connection between being female and taking up the care perspective. This essay refers to the early, and not to the revised, Gilligan views.

Some clarification may be in order to explain why I conferred on Alasdair MacIntyre the title of honorary woman, when to feminists such as Susan Moller Okin[5] he represents a particularly extreme version of patriarchal thinking. It was MacIntyre's anti-Kantian writings that made me regard him as an ally, and also his nostalgia for a virtues-centered variant of ethics. But I agree with Okin that his increasingly explicit defense of a patriarchal religious tradition does make the honor that I did him look undeserved.

Notes

1 Carol Gilligan, *In a Different Voice: Psychological Theory and Women's Development* (Cambridge, Mass.: Harvard University Press, 1982).
2 Ian Hacking, "Winner Take Less," a review of *The Evolution of Cooperation* by Robert Axelrod, *New York Review of Books*, vol. 31, June 28, 1984.
3 Carol Gilligan, "The Conquistador and the Dark Continent: Reflections on the Psychology of Love," *Daedalus*, 113 (Summer 1984): 75–95.
4 "Caring about Caring," a response to Harry Frankfurt's "What We Care About," both in "Matters of the Mind," *Synthese*, 53 (November 1982): 257–90. My paper is also included in my *Postures of the Mind: Essays on Mind and Morals* (Minneapolis, Minn.: University of Minnesota Press, 1985).
5 Susan Moller Okin, *Justice, Gender, and Family* (New York: Basic Books, 1989), esp. chap. 3.

8

Normative Virtue Ethics

Rosalind Hursthouse

A common belief concerning virtue ethics is that it does not tell us what we should do. This belief is sometimes manifested merely in the expressed assumption that virtue ethics, in being 'agent-centred' rather than 'act-centred', is concerned with Being rather than Doing, with good (and bad) character rather than right (and wrong) action, with the question 'What sort of person should I be?' rather than the question 'What should I do?' On this assumption, 'virtue ethics' so-called does not figure as a normative rival to utilitarian and deontological ethics; rather, its (fairly) recent revival is seen as having served the useful purpose of reminding moral philosophers that the elaboration of a normative theory may fall short of giving a full account of our moral life. Thus prompted, deontologists have turned to Kant's long neglected 'Doctrine of Virtue', and utilitarians, largely abandoning the old debate about rule- and act-utilitarianism, are showing interest in the general-happiness-maximizing consequences of inculcating such virtues as friendship, honesty, and loyalty.

On this assumption, it seems that philosophers who 'do virtue ethics', having served this purpose, must realize that they have been doing no more than supplementing normative theory, and should now decide which of the two standard views they espouse. Or, if they find that too difficult, perhaps they should confine themselves to writing detailed studies of particular virtues and vices, indicating where appropriate that 'a deontologist would say that an agent with virtue X will characteristically . . . , whereas a utilitarian would say that she will characteristically . . .' But anyone who wants to espouse virtue ethics as a

Rosalind Hursthouse, "Normative Virtue Ethics," *How Should One Live?* ed. Roger Crisp (Oxford: Clarendon Press, 1996), pp. 19–36.

rival to deontological or utilitarian ethics (finding it distinctly bizarre to suppose that Aristotle espoused either of the latter) will find this common belief voiced against her as an objection: 'Virtue ethics does not, because it cannot, tell us what we should do. Hence it cannot be a normative rival to deontology and utilitarianism.'

This paper is devoted to defending virtue ethics against this objection.

1. Right Action

What grounds might someone have for believing that virtue ethics cannot tell us what we should do? It seems that sometimes the ground is no more than the claim that virtue ethics is concerned with good (and bad) character rather right (and wrong) action. But that claim does no more than highlight an interesting contrast between virtue ethics on the one hand, and deontology and utilitarianism on the other; the former is agent-centred, the latter (it is said) are act-centred.[1] It does not entail that virtue ethics has nothing to say about the concept of right action, nor about which actions are right and which wrong. Wishing to highlight a different contrast, the one between utilitarianism and deontology, we might equally well say, 'Utilitarianism is concerned with good (and bad) states of affairs rather than right (and wrong) action', and no one would take that to mean that utilitarianism, unlike deontology, had nothing to say about right action, for what utilitarianism does say is so familiar.

Suppose an act-utilitarian laid out her account of right action as follows:

U1.   An action is right iff it promotes the best consequences.

This premiss provides a specification of right action, forging the familiar utilitarian link between the concepts of *right action* and *best consequences*, but gives one no guidance about how to act until one knows what to count as the best consequences. So these must be specified in a second premiss, for example:

U2.   The best consequences are those in which happiness is maximized,

which forges the familiar utilitarian link between the concepts of *best consequences* and *happiness*.[2]

Many different versions of deontology can be laid out in a way that displays the same basic structure. They begin with a premiss providing a specification of right action:

D1.   An action is right iff it is in accordance with a correct moral rule or principle.

Like the first premiss of act-utilitarianism, this gives one no guidance about how to act until, in this case, one knows what to count as a correct moral rule (or principle). So this must be specified in a second premiss which begins

D2.   A correct moral rule (principle) is one that . . . ,

and this may be completed in a variety of ways, for example:

(i)   is on the following list (and then a list does follow)
or
(ii)   is laid on us by God
or
(iii)   is universalizable
or
(iv)   would be the object of choice of all rational beings and so on.

Although this way of laying out fairly familiar versions of utilitarianism and deontology is hardly controversial, it is worth noting that it suggests some infelicity in the slogan 'Utilitarianism begins with (or takes as its fundamental concept etc.) the Good, whereas deontology begins with the Right.' If the concept a normative ethics 'begins with' is the one it uses to specify right action, then utilitarianism might be said to begin with the Good (if we take this to be the 'same' concept as that of the *best*), but we should surely hasten to add 'but only in relation to consequences; not, for instance, in relation to *good* agents, or to living *well*'. And even then, we shall not be able to go on to say that most versions of deontology 'begin with' the Right, for they use the concept of moral rule or principle to specify right action. The only versions which, in this sense, 'begin with' the Right would have to be versions of what Frankena calls 'extreme act-deontology',[3] which (I suppose) specify a right action as one which just *is* right.

And if the dictum is supposed to single out, rather vaguely, the concept which is 'most important', then the concepts of *consequences* or *happiness* seem as deserving of mention as the concept of the Good for utilitarianism, and what counts as most important (if any one concept does) for deontologists would surely vary from case to case. For some it would be God, for others universalizability, for others the Categorical Imperative, for others rational acceptance, and so on.

It is possible that too slavish an acceptance of this slogan, and the inevitable difficulty of finding a completion of 'and virtue ethics begins with . . .' which does not reveal its inadequacy, has contributed to the belief that virtue ethics cannot provide a specification of right action. I have heard people say, 'Utilitarianism defines the Right in terms of the Good, and deontology defines the Good in terms of the Right; but how can virtue ethics possibly define both in terms of the (virtuous) Agent?', and indeed, with no answer forthcoming to the questions 'Good *what*? Right *what*?', I have no idea. But if the question is 'How can virtue ethics specify right action?', the answer is easy:

> V1. An action is right iff it is what a virtuous agent would char-
> acteristically (i.e. acting in character) do in the circumstances.

This specification rarely, if ever, silences those who maintain that virtue ethics cannot tell us what we should do. On the contrary, it tends to provoke irritable laughter and scorn. '*That*'s no use', the objectors say. 'It gives us no guidance whatsoever. Who are the virtuous agents?' But if the failure of the first premiss of a normative ethics which forges a link between the concept of right action and a concept distinctive of that ethics may provoke scorn because it provides no practical guidance, why not direct a similar scorn at the first premisses of act-utilitarianism and deontology in the form in which I have given them? Of each of them I remarked, apparently *en passant* but with intent, that they gave us no guidance. Utilitarianism must specify what are to count as the best consequences, and deontology what is to count as a correct moral rule, producing a second premiss, before any guidance is given. And similarly, virtue ethics must specify who is to count as a virtuous agent. So far, the three are all in the same position.

Of course, if the virtuous agent can only be specified as an agent disposed to act in accordance with moral rules, as some have assumed, then virtue ethics collapses back into deontology and is no rival to it. So let us add a subsidiary premiss to this skeletal outline, with the intention of making it clear that virtue ethics aims to provide a non-deontological specification of the virtuous agent via a specification of the virtues, which will be given in its second premiss:

> V1a.   A virtuous agent is one who acts virtuously, that is, one who has and exercises the virtues.
>
> V2.   A virtue is a character trait that . . .[4]

This second premiss of virtue ethics might, like the second premiss of some versions of deontology, be completed simply by enumeration ('a virtue is one of the following', and then the list is given).[5] Or we might, not implausibly, interpret the Hume of the second *Enquiry* as espousing virtue ethics. According to him, a virtue is a character trait (of human beings) that is useful or agreeable to its possessor or to others (inclusive 'or' both times). The standard neo-Aristotelian completion claims that a virtue is a character trait a human being needs for *eudaimonia*, to flourish or live well.

Here, then, we have a specification of right action, whose structure closely resembles those of act-utilitarianism and many forms of deontology. Given that virtue ethics can come up with such a specification, can it still be maintained that it, unlike utilitarianism and deontology, cannot tell us what we should do? Does the specification somehow fail to provide guidance in a way that the other two do not?

At this point, the difficulty of identifying the virtuous agent in a way that makes V1 action-guiding tends to be brought forward again. Suppose it is granted that deontology has just as much difficulty in identifying the correct moral rules as virtue ethics has in identifying the virtues and hence the virtuous agent. Then the following objection may be made.

'All the same,' it may be said, 'if we imagine that that has been achieved – perhaps simply by enumeration – deontology yields a set of clear prescriptions which are readily applicable ("Do not lie", "Do not steal", "Do not inflict evil or harm on others", "Do help others", "Do keep promises", etc.). But virtue ethics yields only the prescription "Do what the virtuous agent (the one who is honest, charitable, just, etc.) would do in these circumstances." And this gives me no guidance unless I am (and know I am) a virtuous agent myself (in which case I am hardly in need of it). If I am less than fully virtuous, I shall have no idea what a virtuous agent would do, and hence cannot apply the only prescription that virtue ethics has given me. (Of course, act-utilitarianism also yields a single prescription, "Do what maximises happiness", but there are no *parallel* difficulties in applying that.) So there is the way in which V1 fails to be action-guiding where deontology and utilitarianism succeed.'

It is worth pointing out that, if I acknowledge that I am far from perfect, and am quite unclear what a virtuous agent would do in the circumstances in which I find myself, the obvious thing to do is to go and ask one, should this be possible. This is far from being a trivial point, for it gives a straightforward explanation of an aspect of our moral life which should not be ignored, namely the fact that we do seek moral guidance from people who we think are morally better than ourselves. When I am looking for an excuse to do something I have a horrid suspicion is wrong, I ask my moral inferiors (or peers if I am bad enough), 'Wouldn't you do such and such if you were in my shoes?' But when I am anxious to do what is right, and do not see my way clear, I go to people I respect and admire – people who I think are kinder, more honest, more just, wiser, than I am myself – and ask them what they would do in my circumstances. How utilitarianism and deontology would explain this fact, I do not know; but, as I said, the explanation within the terms of virtue ethics is straightforward. If you want to do what is right, and doing what is right is doing what a virtuous agent would do in the circumstances, then you should find out what she would do if you do not already know.

Moreover, seeking advice from virtuous people is not the only thing an imperfect agent trying to apply the single prescription of virtue ethics can do. For it is simply false that, in general, 'if I am less than fully virtuous, then I shall have no idea what a virtuous agent would do', as the objection claims. Recall that we are assuming that the virtues have been enumerated, as the deontologist's rules have been. The latter have been enumerated as, say, 'Do not lie', 'Do not inflict evil or harm', etc.; the former as, say, honesty, charity, justice, etc. So, *ex hypothesi*, a virtuous agent is one who is honest, charitable, just, etc. So what she characteristically does is act honestly, charitably, justly, etc., and not dishonestly, uncharitably, unjustly. So given an enumeration of the virtues, I may well have a perfectly good idea of what the virtuous person would do in my circumstances despite my own imperfection. Would she lie in her teeth to acquire an unmerited advantage? No, for that would be to act both dishonestly and unjustly. Would she help the naked man by the roadside or pass by on the other side? The former, for she acts charitably. Might she keep a deathbed promise even though living people would benefit from its being broken? Yes, for she acts justly.[6] And so on.

2.   Moral Rules

The above response to the objection that V1 fails to be action-guiding clearly amounts to a denial of the oft-repeated claim that virtue ethics does not come up with any rules (another version of the thought that it is concerned with Being rather than Doing and needs to be supplemented with rules). We can now see that it comes up with a large number; not only does each virtue generate a prescription – act honestly, charitably, justly – but each vice a prohibition – do not act dishonestly, uncharitably, unjustly. Once this point about virtue ethics is grasped (and it is remarkable how often it is overlooked), can there remain any reason for thinking that virtue ethics cannot tell us what we should do? Yes. The reason given is, roughly, that rules such as 'Act honestly', 'Do not act uncharitably', etc. are, like the rule 'Do what the virtuous agent would do', still the wrong sort of rule, still somehow doomed to fail to provide the action guidance supplied by the rules (or rule) of deontology and utilitarianism.

But how so? It is true that these rules of virtue ethics (henceforth 'v-rules') are couched in terms, or concepts, which are certainly 'evaluative' in *some* sense, or senses, of that difficult word. Is it this which dooms them to failure? Surely not, unless many forms of deontology fail too.[7] If we concentrate on the single example of lying, defining lying to be 'asserting what you believe to be untrue, with the intention of deceiving your hearer(s)', then we might, for a moment, preserve the illusion that a deontologist's rules do not contain 'evaluative' terms.[8] But as soon as we remember that few deontologists will want to forgo principles of non-maleficence or beneficence, the illusion vanishes. For those principles, and their corresponding rules ('Do no evil or harm to others', 'Help others', 'Promote their well-being'), rely on terms or concepts which are at least as 'evaluative' as those employed in the v-rules.[9] Few deontologists rest content with the simple quasi-biological 'Do not kill', but more refined versions of that rule such as 'Do not murder', or 'Do not kill the innocent', once again employ 'evaluative' terms, and 'Do not kill unjustly' is itself a particular instantiation of a v-rule.

Supposing this point were granted, a deontologist might still claim that the v-rules are markedly inferior to deontological rules as far as providing guidance for children is concerned. Granted, adult deontologists must think hard about what really constitutes harming someone, or promoting their well-being, or respecting their autonomy, or murder, but surely the simple rules we learnt at our mother's knee are indispensable? How could virtue ethics plausibly seek to dispense with these and expect toddlers to grasp 'Act charitably, honestly, and kindly', 'Don't act unjustly', and so on? Rightly are these concepts described as 'thick'![10] Far too thick for a child to grasp.

Strictly speaking, this claim about learning does not really support the *general* claim that v-rules fail to provide action-guidance, but the claim about learning, arising naturally as it does in the context of the general claim, is one I am more than happy to address. For it pinpoints a condition of adequacy that any normative ethics must meet, namely that such an ethics must not only come up with action-guidance for a clever rational adult but also generate some account of moral education, of how one generation teaches the next what they should do. But an ethics inspired by Aristotle is unlikely to have forgotten the question of moral education, and the objection fails to hit home. First, the implicit empirical claim that toddlers are taught *only* the deontologist's rules, not the 'thick' concepts, is false. Sentences such as 'Don't do that, it hurts, you mustn't be *cruel*', 'Be *kind* to your brother, he's only little', 'Don't be so *mean*, so *greedy*' are commonly addressed to toddlers. Secondly, why should a proponent of virtue ethics deny the significance of such mother's-knee rules as 'Don't lie', 'Keep promises', 'Don't take more than your fair share', 'Help others'? Although it is a mistake, I have claimed, to define a virtuous agent simply as one disposed to act in accordance with moral rules, it is a very understandable mistake, given the obvious connection between, for example, the exercise of the virtue of honesty and refraining from lying. Virtue ethicists want to emphasize the fact that, if children are to be taught to be honest, they must be taught to prize the truth, and that *merely* teaching them not to lie will not achieve this end. But they need not deny that to achieve this end teaching them not to lie is useful, even indispensable.

So we can see that virtue ethics not only comes up with rules (the v-rules, couched in terms derived from the virtues and vices), but further, does not exclude the more familiar deontologists' rules. The theoretical distinction between the two is that the familiar rules, and their applications in particular cases, are given entirely different backings. According to virtue ethics, I must not tell this lie, since it would be dishonest, and dishonesty is a vice; must not break this promise, since it would be unjust, or a betrayal of friendship, or, perhaps (for the available virtue and vice terms do not neatly cover every contingency), simply because no virtuous person would.

However, the distinction is not merely theoretical. It is, indeed, the case that, with respect to a number of familiar examples, virtue ethicists and deontologists tend to stand shoulder to shoulder against utilitarians, denying that, for example, this lie can be told, this promise broken, this human being killed because the consequences of so doing will be generally happiness-maximizing. But, despite a fair amount of coincidence in action-guidance between deontology and virtue ethics, the latter has its own distinctive approach to the practical problems involved in dilemmas.

3.   The Conflict Problem

It is a noteworthy fact that, in support of the general claim that virtue ethics cannot tell us what we should do, what is often cited is the 'conflict problem'. The requirements of different virtues, it is said, can point us in opposed directions. Charity prompts me to kill the person who would (truly) be better off dead, but justice forbids it. Honesty points to telling the hurtful truth, kindness and compassion to remaining silent or even lying. And so on. So virtue ethics lets us down just at the point where we need it, where we are faced with the really difficult dilemmas and do not know what to do.

In the mouth of a utilitarian, this may be a comprehensible criticism, for, as is well known, the only conflict that classical utilitarianism's one rule can generate is the tiresome logical one between the two occurrences of 'greatest' in its classical statement. But it is strange to find the very same criticism coming from deontologists, who are notoriously faced with the same problem. 'Don't kill', 'Respect autonomy', 'Tell the truth', 'Keep promises' may all conflict with 'Prevent suffering' or 'Do no harm', which is precisely why deontologists so often reject utilitarianism's deliverances on various dilemmas. Presumably, they must think that deontology can solve the 'conflict problem' and, further, that virtue ethics cannot. Are they right?

With respect to a number of cases, the deontologist's strategy is to argue that the 'conflict' is merely apparent, or *prima facie*. The proponent of virtue ethics employs the same strategy: according to her, many of the putative conflicts are merely apparent, resulting from a misapplication of the virtue or vice terms. Does kindness require not telling hurtful truths? Sometimes, but in *this* case, what has to be understood is that one does people no kindness by concealing this sort of truth from them, hurtful as it may be. Or, in a different case, the importance of the truth in question puts the consideration of hurt feelings out of court, and the agent does not show herself to be unkind, or callous, by speaking out. Does charity require that I kill the person who would be better off dead but who wants to stay alive, thereby conflicting with justice? Not if, in Foot's words, '[a] man does not lack charity because he refrains from an act of injustice which would have been for someone's good'.[11]

One does not have to agree with the three judgements expressed here to recognize this as a *strategy* available to virtue ethics, any more than one has to agree with the particular judgements of deontologists who, for example, may claim that one rule outranks another, or that a certain rule has a certain exception clause built in, when they argue that a putative case of conflict is resolvable. Whether an individual has resolved a putative moral conflict or dilemma rightly is one question; whether a normative ethics has the wherewithal to resolve it is an entirely different question, and it is the latter with which we are concerned here.

The form the strategy takes within virtue ethics provides what may plausibly be claimed to be the deep explanation of why, in some cases, agents do not know the answer to 'What should I do in these circumstances?' despite the fact that there *is* an answer. Trivially, the explanation is that they lack moral knowledge of what to do in this situation; but why? In what way? The lack, according to virtue ethics' strategy, arises from lack of moral wisdom, from an inadequate grasp of what is involved in acting *kindly* (unkindly) or *charitably* (uncharitably), in being *honest*, or *just*, or *lacking in charity*, or, in general, of how the virtue (and vice) terms are to be correctly applied.

Here we come to an interesting defence of the v-rules, often criticized as being too difficult to apply for the agent who lacks moral wisdom.[12] The defence relies on an (insufficiently acknowledged) insight of Aristotle's – namely that moral knowledge, unlike mathematical knowledge, cannot be acquired merely by attending lectures and is not characteristically to be found in people too young to have much experience of life.[13] Now *if* right action were determined by rules that any clever adolescent could apply correctly, how could this be so? Why are there not moral whiz-kids, the way there are mathematical (or quasi-mathematical) whiz-kids? But if the rules that determine right action are, like the v-rules, very difficult to apply correctly, involving, for instance, a grasp of the *sort* of truth that one does people no kindness by concealing, the explanation is readily to hand. Clever adolescents do not, in general, have a good grasp of that sort of thing.[14] And *of course* I have to say 'the sort of truth that . . .' and 'that sort of thing', relying on my readers' knowledgeable uptake. For if I could define either sort, then, once again, clever adolescents could acquire moral wisdom from textbooks.

So far, I have described one strategy available to virtue ethics for coping with the 'conflict problem', a strategy that consists in arguing that the conflict is merely apparent, and can be resolved. According to one – only one of many – versions of 'the doctrine of the unity of the virtues', this is the only possible strategy (and ultimately successful), but this is not a claim I want to defend. One general reason is that I still do not know what I think about 'the unity of the virtues' (all those different versions!); a more particular, albeit related, reason is that, even if I were (somehow) sure that the requirements of the particular virtues could never conflict, I suspect that I would still believe in the possibility of moral dilemmas. I have been talking so far as though examples of putative dilemmas and examples of putative conflict between the requirements of different virtues (or deontologists' rules) coincided. But it may seem to many, as it does to me, that there are certain (putative) dilemmas which can only be described in terms of (putative) conflict with much artifice and loss of relevant detail.

Let us, therefore, consider the problem of moral dilemmas without bothering about whether they can be described in the simple terms of a conflict between the requirements of two virtues (or two deontologists' rules). Most of us, it may be supposed, have our own favoured example(s), either real or imaginary, of the case (or cases) where we see the decision about whether to do A or B as a very grave matter, have thought a great deal about what can be said for and against doing A, and doing B, and have still not managed to reach a conclusion which we think is the right one.[15] How, if at all, does virtue ethics direct us to think about such cases?

4.   Dilemmas and Normative Theory

As a preliminary to answering that question, we should consider a much more general one, namely 'How should any normative ethics direct us to think about such cases?' This brings us to the topic of normative theory.

It is possible to detect a new movement in moral philosophy, a movement which has already attracted the name 'anti-theory in ethics'.[16] Its various representatives have as a common theme the rejection of normative ethical theory; but amongst them are numbered several philosophers usually associated with virtue ethics, such as Baier, McDowell, MacIntyre, and Nussbaum. This does not mean that they maintain what I have been denying, namely that virtue ethics is not normative; rather, they assume that it does not constitute a normative *theory* (and, mindful of this fact, I have been careful to avoid describing virtue ethics as one). What is meant by a 'normative theory' in this context is not easy to pin down, but, roughly, a normative theory is taken to be a set (possibly one-membered in the case of utilitarianism) of general principles which provide a *decision procedure* for all questions about how to act morally.

Part of the point of distinguishing a normative ethics by calling it a normative 'theory' is that a decent theory, as we know from science, enables us to answer questions that we could not answer before we had it. It is supposed to resolve those difficult dilemmas in which, it is said, our moral intuitions clash, and, prior to our grasp of the theory, we do not know what we should do.[17] And a large part of the motivation for subscribing to 'anti-theory in ethics' is the belief that we should not be looking to science to provide us with our model of moral knowledge. Our 'intuitions' in ethics do not play the same role *vis-à-vis* the systematic articulation of moral knowledge as our 'observations' play *vis-à-vis* the systematic articulation of scientific knowledge; many of the goals appropriate to scientific knowledge – universality, consistency, completeness, simplicity – are not appropriate to moral knowledge; the acquisition of moral knowledge involves the training of the emotions in a way that the acquisition of scientific knowledge does not; and so on.

Clearly, many different issues are involved in the question of the extent to which moral knowledge should be modelled on scientific knowledge. The one I want to focus on here is the issue of whether a normative ethics should provide a decision procedure which enables us to resolve all moral dilemmas. Should it, to rephrase the question I asked above, (1) direct us to think about moral dilemmas in the belief that they *must* have a resolution, and that it is the business of the normative ethics in question to provide one? Or should it (2) have built into it the possibility of there being, as David Wiggins puts it, some 'absolutely undecidable questions – e.g. cases where . . . nothing could count as *the* reasonable practical answer',[18] counting questions about dilemmas of the sort described as amongst them? Or should it (3) be sufficiently flexible to allow for a comprehensible disagreement on this issue between two proponents of the normative ethics in question?

If we are to avoid modelling normative ethics mindlessly on scientific theory, we should not simply assume that the first position is the correct one. But rejection of such a model is not enough to justify the second position either. Someone might believe that for *any* dilemma there must be something that counts as the right way out of it, without believing that normative ethics remotely resembles scientific theory, perhaps because they subscribe to a version of realism (in Dummett's sense of 'realism').[19]

More particularly, someone might believe on religious grounds that if I find myself, through no fault of my own, confronted with a dilemma (of the sort described), there must be something that counts as the right way out of it.[20] The belief in God's providence does indeed involve, as Geach says, the thought that 'God does not require of a faithful servant the desperate choice between sin and sin.'[21] Should a normative ethics be such that it cannot be shared by a realist and an anti-realist (again in Dummett's sense)? Or by an atheist and a theist? It seems to me that a normative ethics should be able to accommodate such differences, and so I subscribe to the third position outlined above.

Which position utilitarians and deontologists might espouse is not my concern here; I want to make clear how it is that virtue ethics is able to accommodate the third.[22]

Let us return to V1 – 'An action is right iff it is what a virtuous agent would characteristically do in the circumstances.' This makes it clear that if two people disagree about the possibility of irresolvable moral dilemmas, their disagreement will manifest itself in what they say about the virtue of agents. So let us suppose that two candidates for being virtuous agents are each faced with their own case of the same dilemma. (I do not want to defend the view that each situation is unique in such a way that nothing would count as two agents being in the same circumstances and faced with the same dilemma.) And, after much thought, one does A and the other does B.

Now, those who believe that there cannot be irresolvable dilemmas (of the sort described) can say that, in the particular case, at least one agent, say the one who did A, thereby showed themselves to be lacking in virtue, perhaps in that practical wisdom which is an essential aspect of each of the 'non-intellectual' virtues. ('If you can *see* no way out but a lie, the lie may be the least wicked of the alternatives you can discern: it is still wicked, and you should blame yourself that you lacked the wisdom of St. Joan or St. Athanasius, to extricate yourself without lying. It is not a matter of foxy cleverness; "the testimony of the LORD is sure and giveth wisdom to the simple".'[23] Thus Geach, discussing the absolute prohibition against lying in the context of the claim that God 'does not require of any man a choice between sin and sin'.) Or they can say that at least one agent must have been lacking in virtue, without claiming to know which.

But those who believe that there are, or may be, irresolvable dilemmas can suppose that both agents are not merely candidates for being, but actually are, virtuous agents. For to believe in such dilemmas is to believe in cases in which even the perfect practical wisdom that the most idealized virtuous agent has does not direct her to do, say, A rather than

B. And then the fact that these virtuous agents acted differently, despite being in the same circumstances, *determines* the fact that there is no answer to the question 'What is *the* right thing to do in these circumstances?' For if it is true both that *a* virtuous agent would do A, and that *a* virtuous agent would do B (as it is, since, *ex hypothesi*, one did do A and the other B), then both A and B are, in the circumstances, right, according to V1.

The acceptance of this should not be taken as a counsel of despair, nor as an excuse for moral irresponsibility. It does not license coin-tossing when one is faced with a putative dilemma, for the moral choices we find most difficult do not come to us conveniently labelled as 'resolvable' or 'irresolvable'. I was careful to specify that the two candidates for being virtuous agents acted only 'after much thought'. It will always be necessary to think very hard before accepting the idea that a particular moral decision does not have one right issue, and, even on the rare occasions on which she eventually reached the conclusion that this is such a case, would the virtuous agent toss a coin? Of course not.

No doubt someone will say, 'Well, if she really thinks the dilemma is irresolvable, why not, according to virtue ethics?', and the answer must, I think, be *ad hominem*. If their conception of the virtuous agent – of someone with the character traits of justice, honesty, compassion, kindness, loyalty, wisdom, etc. – really is of someone who would resort to coin-tossing when confronted with what she believed to be an irresolvable dilemma, then that is the bizarre conception they bring to virtue ethics, and they must, presumably, think that there is nothing morally irresponsible or light-minded about coin-tossing in such cases. So they should not want virtue ethics to explain 'why not'. But if their conception of the virtuous agent does not admit of her acting thus – if they think such coin-tossing would be irresponsible, or light-minded, or indeed simply insane – then they have no need to ask the question. *My* question was, 'Would the virtuous agent toss a coin?'; they agree that of course she would not. Why not? Because it would be irresponsible, or light-minded, or the height of folly.

The acceptance of the possibility of irresolvable dilemmas within virtue ethics (by those of us who do accept it) should not be seen in itself as conceding much to 'pluralism'. If I say that I can imagine a case in which two virtuous agents are faced with a dilemma, and one does A while the other does B, I am not saying that I am imagining a case in which the two virtuous agents each think that what the other does is wrong (vicious, contrary to virtue) because they have radically different views about what is required by a certain virtue, or about whether a certain character trait is a vice, or about whether something is to be greatly valued or of little importance. I am imagining a case in which my two virtuous agents have the same 'moral views' about everything, up to and including the view that, in this particular case, neither decision is *the* right one, and hence neither is wrong. Each recognizes the propriety of the other's reason for doing what she did – say, 'To avoid *that* evil', 'To secure *this* good' – for her recognition of the fact that this is as good a moral reason as her own (say, 'To avoid *this* evil', 'To secure *that* good') is what forced each to accept the idea that the dilemma was irresolvable in the first place. Though each can give such a reason for what they did (A in one case, B in the other), neither attempts to give 'the moral reason' why they did one *rather than* the other. The 'reason' for or explanation of *that* would be, if available at all, in terms of psychological autobiography ('I decided to sleep on it, and when I woke up I just found myself thinking in terms of doing A', or 'I just felt terrified at the thought of doing A: I'm sure this was totally irrational, but I did, so I did B').[24]

The topic of this chapter has been the view that virtue ethics cannot be a normative rival to utilitarianism and deontology because 'it cannot tell us what we should do'. In defending the existence of normative virtue ethics I have not attempted to argue that it can 'tell us what we should do' in such a way that the difficult business of acting well is made easy for us. I have not only admitted but welcomed the fact that, in some cases, moral wisdom is required if the v-rules are to be applied correctly and apparent dilemmas thereby resolved (or indeed identified, since a choice that may seem quite straightforward to the foolish or wicked may rightly appear difficult, calling for much thought, to the wise). Nor have I attempted to show that virtue ethics is guaranteed to be able to resolve every dilemma. It seems bizarre to insist that a normative ethics must be able to do this prior to forming a reasonable belief that there cannot be irresolvable dilemmas, but those who have formed such a belief may share a normative ethics with those who have different views concerning realism, or the existence of God. A normative ethics, I suggested, should be able to accommodate both views on this question, as virtue ethics does, not model itself mindlessly on scientific theory.[25]

Notes

1   Kant is standardly taken as the paradigm deontologist, but Stephen Hudson argues he is much closer to Aristotle on the act/agent-centred point than is usually supposed. See 'What is Morality All About?', *Philosophia* 20 (1990), 3–13.

2 Variations on utilitarianism are not my concern here. I am ignoring rule-utilitarianism, and assuming my reader to be well aware of the fact that different utilitarians may specify *best consequences* in different ways. See the introduction to A. Sen and B. Williams (eds.), *Utilitarianism and Beyond* (Cambridge, 1982), from which I have (basically) taken the characterization of utilitarianism given here.

3 W. Frankena, *Ethics*, 2nd edn. (Englewood Cliffs, NJ, 1973), 16.

4 It might be said that V1a does not make it clear that virtue ethics aims to provide a non-deontological specification of the virtuous agent, since it does not rule out the possibility that the virtues themselves are no more than dispositions to act in accordance with moral rules. And indeed, it does seem that the belief that the virtuous agent is nothing but the agent disposed to act in accordance with moral rules is often based on that assumption about the virtues. (See, for example, Frankena, *Ethics*, 65 and A. Gewirth, 'Rights and Virtues', *Review of Metaphysics* 38 (1985), 739–62.) Then we must say that V2 aims to clear that up by saying that the virtues are character traits, assuming it to be obvious that someone's being of a certain character is not merely a matter of her being disposed to do certain sorts of acts in accordance with a rule.

5 'Enumeration' may connote something more explicit than is required. Deontologists and virtue ethicists actually engaged in normative ethics may well do no more than take it as obvious in the course of what they say that such-and-such is a correct moral rule or virtue, neither stipulating this explicitly, nor attempting to list other rules/virtues which have no bearing on whatever issue is under discussion.

6 I follow tradition here in taking the virtue of fidelity, or faithfulness to one's word, to be part of the virtue of justice, thereby avoiding a clumsy attempt to manufacture an adverbial phrase corresponding to 'fidelity'. But nothing hangs on this.

7 Forms of utilitarianism which aim to be entirely value-free or empirical, such as those which define happiness in terms of the satisfaction of actual desires or preferences, regardless of their content, or as a mental state whose presence is definitively established by introspection, seem to me the least plausible, but I accept that anyone who embraces them may consistently complain that v-rules give inferior action-guidance in virtue of containing 'evaluative' terms. But any utilitarian who wishes to employ any distinction between the higher and lower pleasures, or rely on some list of goods (such as autonomy, friendship, knowledge of important matters) in defining happiness, must grant that even her single rule is implicitly 'evaluative'.

8 It might be thought that the example of promises provided an equally straightforward example. This would not substantially affect my argument, but in any case, I do not think that this is so. The *Shorter Oxford* defines the verb 'to promise' as 'to undertake or . . . , by word or . . . , to do or refrain . . . , or to give . . . : usu. to the *advantage* of the person concerned' (my italics),

and the qualification containing the word I have italicized seems to me essential. Its significance has been highlighted in the many stories and myths whose tragic point turns on someone wicked doing what they literally undertook to do, to the horror and despair of 'the person concerned'. ('Promise me you will fearfully punish the one who has done so and so', the person concerned says, not realizing that the one in question is her long-lost son.)

9   I cannot resist pointing out that this reveals a further inadequacy in the slogan 'Utilitarianism begins with the Good, deontology with the Right' when this is taken as committing deontology to making the concept of the Good (and presumably the Bad or Evil) somehow derivative from the concept of the Right (and Wrong). A 'utilitarian' who relied on the concept of *morally right*, or *virtuous*, action in specifying his concept of happiness would find it hard to shrug off the scare quotes, but no one expects a deontologist to be able to state each of her rules without employing a concept of *good* which is not simply the concept of *right action for its own sake*, or without any mention of *evil* or *harm*.

10   See B. Williams, *Ethics and the Limits of Philosophy* (London, 1985), 129–30.

11   P. Foot, *Virtues and Vices* (Oxford, 1978), p. 60, n. 12.

12   This could well be regarded as another version of the criticism discussed earlier, that the v-rules somehow fail to provide action-guidance.

13   *Nicomachean Ethics* (= NE) 1142^{a}12–16.

14   In defending the thesis that virtue ethics is a normative *rival* to utilitarianism and deontology, I am not simultaneously aiming to establish the far more ambitious thesis that it beats its rivals hollow. Utilitarians and deontologists may well take the Aristotelian point on board and provide an account, appropriate to their ethics, of why we should not consult whiz-kids about difficult moral decisions. For example, Onora O'Neill's sophisticated version of Kantian 'maxims' rules out their application by (merely) clever adolescents.

15   I have chosen this description of the sort of dilemmas with which I am concerned deliberately, mindful of Philippa Foot's paper, 'Moral Realism and Moral Dilemma', *The Journal of Philosophy* 80 (1983), 379–98. As she points out, some cases that are discussed as 'conflicts' or 'dilemmas' are taken to be resolvable, that is, taken to be cases in which we do reach a conclusion we think is the right one; these are my cases of 'apparent' conflict. Commenting on Wiggins (see below, n. 18), she also points out that undecidability may exist 'in small moral matters, or where the choice is between goods rather than evils, only it doesn't worry us' (395); I am concentrating on the ones that worry us.

16   See S. Clarke and E. Simpson (eds.), *Anti-Theory in Ethics and Moral Conservatism* (New York, 1989), containing, *inter alia*, articles by Baier, McDowell, MacIntyre, and Nussbaum, as well as Cheryl N. Noble's seminal 'Normative Ethical Theories' (49–64). It is noteworthy that, in the latter, Noble

explicitly denies that she is attacking the idea of normative *ethics*. Her criticisms of the idea of normative ethical *theory*, she says, 'are aimed at a particular conception of what normative ethics should be' (62, n. 1).

17 As Noble points out, a normative theory may also be expected to say something about cases 'where we have no intuitions or where our intuitions are inchoate or weak' (ibid. 61); and, to some of us, it is indeed one of the oddities of utilitarianism that certain states of affairs, concerning which we may have no moral intuitions at all, emerge from it as so definitively 'morally better' than others. I would like to argue for the incoherence of the idea that a theory could attach a truth-value to a sentence (employing a moral term) which lacked a sense outside the theory, but space does not permit. See, however, P. Foot, 'Utilitarianism and the Virtues', *Mind* 94 (1985), 196–209.

18 D. Wiggins, 'Truth, Invention and the Meaning of Life', *Proceedings of the British Academy* 62 (1976), 371, my italics. I have omitted the phrase that attracted Foot's criticism (see above, n. 15), in which Wiggins seems to imply that undecidable questions are undecidable *because* the alternatives are particularly terrible.

19 M. Dummett, *Truth and Other Enigmas* (London, 1978), 1–24 and 145–65. For a brief but helpful discussion of the distinction between Dummett-type realism and cognitivism in ethics, see Foot, 'Moral Realism and Moral Dilemma', 397–8.

20 I am assuming that the qualification 'through no fault of my own' is all-important, since I cannot imagine why anyone should think (except through oversight) that there must always be a right action I can do to get myself out of any mess that I have got myself into through previous wrongdoing.

21 P. Geach, *The Virtues* (Cambridge, 1977), 155.

22 I had hitherto overlooked the possibility of this third position, and hence had emphasized the fact that virtue ethics could occupy the second. But I subsequently heard Philippa Foot point out that Aquinas, Anscombe, and Geach should surely be classified as virtue ethicists, notwithstanding their absolutist stance on many of the familiar deontological rules; and, given their consequent stance on the clear resolvability of some dilemmas that others find irresolvable, this prompted me to look at what a commitment to resolvability (with respect to dilemmas *as described*) might look like within virtue ethics. I am grateful to the editor for reminding me of the further possibility of his own 'realist' position. (Aristotle is clearly an absolutist too, at least with respect to 'adultery' (*moikheia*), theft, and murder (see *NE* 1107[a]11–12), but where he stands (or should stand, to be consistent) on irresolvable dilemmas of the sort described is, I think, entirely unclear.)

23 Geach, *The Virtues*, 121.

24 It must be remembered that, *ex hypothesi*, these are things said by virtuous agents about what they did when confronted with an irresolvable dilemma. Of course they would be very irresponsible accounts of why one had done A rather than B in a resolvable case.

25   At the request of the editor, I have repeated here several points I have made in two other papers, 'Virtue Theory and Abortion', *Philosophy and Public Affairs* 20 (1991), 223–46, and 'Applying Virtue Ethics', in *Virtues and Reasons: Philippa Foot and Moral Theory*, ed. R. Hursthouse, G. Lawrence, and W. S. Quinn (Oxford, 1995), 57–75.

9

Agent-Based Virtue Ethics

Michael Slote

A tremendous revival of interest in virtue ethics has recently been taking place, but in this paper I would like to discuss some important virtue-ethical possibilities that have yet to be substantially explored. Till now Aristotle has been the principal focus of new interest in virtue ethics, but it is possible to pursue virtue ethics in a more *agent-based* fashion than what we (or some of us) find in Aristotle. I am going to explore that possibility here and attempt to explain why such a more radical approach is not as outré, misconceived, inappropriate, or obviously unpromising as it is sometimes held to be.[1]

1. Agent-Based versus Agent-Focused Virtue Ethics

An agent-based approach to virtue ethics treats the moral or ethical status of acts as entirely derivative from independent and fundamental aretaic (as opposed to deontic) ethical characterizations of motives, character traits, or individuals, and such agent-basing is arguably not to be found in Aristotle, at least on one kind of standard interpretation. To be sure, Aristotle seems to put a greater emphasis on the evaluation of agents and character traits than he does on the evaluation of actions. Moreover, for Aristotle an act is noble or fine if it is one that a noble or virtuous individual would perform, and he does say that the virtuous individual is the measure of virtue in action. But Aristotle also allows that properly guided or momentarily inspired individuals can perform fine or good or virtuous acts even if the individuals are not themselves good or virtuous,

Michael Slote, "Agent-Based Virtue Ethics," *Midwest Studies in Philosophy* 20 (1995): 83–101 (20).

and, in addition, he characterizes the virtuous individual as someone who *sees* or *perceives* what is good or fine or right to do in any given situation.

Such language clearly implies that the virtuous individual does what is noble or virtuous because it is the noble – e.g., courageous – thing to do, rather than its being the case that what is noble – or courageous – to do has this status simply because the virtuous individual will choose or has chosen it. Even if right or fine actions cannot be defined in terms of rules, what makes them right or fine, for Aristotle, is not that they have been chosen in a certain way by a certain sort of individual. So their status as right or fine or noble is treated as in some measure independent of agent-evaluations, and that is incompatible with agent-basing as we defined it just above. (If the virtuous individual is the measure of what is fine or right, that may simply mean that she is in the *best possible position to know or perceive* what is fine or right.)

Thus we must distinguish a virtue-ethical theory like Aristotle's (as commonly interpreted), which focuses more on virtuous individuals and individual traits than on actions and is thus in some sense *agent-focused*, from agent-based views which, unlike Aristotle,[2] treat the moral or ethical status of actions as entirely derivative from independent and fundamental ethical aretaic facts (or claims) about the motives, dispositions, or inner life of the individuals who perform them. Views of the latter kind clearly represent an extreme or radical form of virtue ethics, and indeed it is somewhat difficult to find clear-cut historical examples of such agent-basing. In fact, the only absolutely clear-cut example of agent-basing I have found is that of the nineteenth-century British ethicist James Martineau. Other potential historical examples of agent-basing – notably, Hume, Leslie Stephen, Nietzsche, Abelard, Augustine, and Kant – offer different forms of resistance to such interpretation, and even Plato, who insists that we evaluate actions by reference to the health and virtue of the individual soul, seems to think that appreciation of the Form of the Good represents a level of evaluation prior to the evaluation of souls, with souls counting as virtuous when properly appreciating and being guided by the value inherent in the Form of the Good. To that extent, Plato's view is not agent-*based*, but I believe there is a way of freeing the Platonic approach from dependence on the Forms, and the first form of agent-basing I shall be describing has its ultimate inspiration in Plato. The other ways of agent-basing I shall go on to describe can be seen as more plausible simplifying variants on Martineau's moral theory. But before I say more about particular ways of developing agent-based virtue theories, there are some very worrying objections to the whole idea of agent-basing that must first be addressed.[3]

2. Two Objections to Agent-Basing

One thing that seems wrong in principle with any agent-based approach to moral evaluation is that it appears to obliterate the common distinction between doing the right thing and doing the right thing for the right reasons. Sidgwick's well-known example of the prosecutor who does his duty by trying to convict a defendant, but who is motivated by malice rather than by a sense of duty, seems to illustrate the distinction in question, and it may well seem that agent-based virtue ethics would have difficulty here because of the way it understands rightness in terms of having good motivations and wrongness in terms of having bad motives. If actions are wrong when they result from morally bad motives, does that not mean that the prosecutor does the wrong thing in prosecuting someone out of malice (assuming that malice is morally criticizable in general or in this particular case)? And isn't that a rather unfortunate consequence of the agent-based approach?

I am not sure. Sidgwick himself seems to grant a certain plausibility to the idea that the prosecutor acts wrongly if he prosecutes from malice.[4] What *is* implausible is merely the claim that the prosecutor has no obligation to prosecute, which doesn't follow from the agent-based assumption that he acts wrongly if he prosecutes from malice. Sidgwick of course points out that if he is sufficiently motivated by malice, the prosecutor may be unable to do his duty entirely or even substantially for the right kind of reason. But this merely entails that there is no way the prosecutor who is motivated thus can avoid acting wrongly if he prosecutes. It does not mean it is morally all right for him *not* to prosecute, or thus that he has no duty or obligation to prosecute.

But how can such a duty be understood in agent-based terms? Consider the possibility that *if he does not prosecute,* the prosecutor's motivation will *also* be bad. Those who talk about the malicious prosecutor case often fail to mention the motives that might lead him *not* to prosecute. With malice present or even in the absence of malice, if the prosecutor doesn't prosecute, one very likely explanation will be that he lacks real or strong concern for doing his job and playing the contributing social role which that involves. Imagine, for example, that horrified by his own malice he decides not to prosecute. This too will be motivated by a bad motive, insufficient concern for the public (or general human) good or for making his contribution to society – motives I shall have a good deal more to say about in discussing positive versions of agent-based views.

So the idea that motives are the basis for evaluating actions that they cause or that express them doesn't have particularly untoward results. And it allows us something like the distinction between doing the right thing and doing the right thing for the right reason. In particular, it allows us to say that the prosecutor has a duty to prosecute, because if he does not we shall in the normal course (barring a heart attack, nervous breakdown, religious conversion, and such like) be able to attribute to him motivation, or deficient or defective motivation, of a kind that makes his act wrong. Yet we can also say that if he prosecutes, he acts wrongly, even if another person, with different motivation, would have acted rightly in doing so. This allows us then to distinguish between doing one's duty for the right reasons and thus acting rightly, on the one hand, and doing one's duty for the wrong reasons and thus acting wrongly. This is very close to the distinction between right action and acting rightly for the right reasons, except for the fact it supposes that when the reasons aren't right, the action itself is actually *wrong*. But we have already seen that this idea is not in itself particularly implausible. And what we now see is that the above-mentioned complaint against agent-basing boils down to a faulty assumption about the inability of such views to make fine-grained distinctions of the sort we have just succeeded in making.

However, there is another objection to the whole idea of agent-basing that may more fundamentally represent what seems objectionable and even bizarre about any such approach to morality or ethics. If the evaluation of actions ultimately derives from that of (the inner states of) agents, then it would appear to follow that if one is the right sort of person or possesses the right sort of inner states, it doesn't morally matter what one actually *does*, so that the person, or at least her actions, are subject to no genuine moral requirements or constraints. In this light, agent-basing seems a highly autistic and antinomian approach to ethics, an approach that seems to undermine the familiar, intuitive notion that the moral or ethical life involves, among other things, *living up to* certain *standards* of behavior or action. Such an implication would seem to be totally unacceptable from the standpoint of anyone who takes ethics and the moral life seriously. Indeed, this train of reasoning once caused me to abandon the whole idea of agent-based morality, before I saw that the implications drawn just now do not in fact follow in any way from agent-basing.[5] A view can be agent-based and still not treat actions as right or admirable simply because they are done by a virtuous individual or by someone with an admirable or good inner state. Nor does an agent-based theory have to say, with respect to each and every action a virtuous agent is capable of performing, that if she were to perform that action, it would automatically count as a good or admirable thing for her to have done.

Thus consider a very simple view according to which (roughly) benevolence is the only good motive and acts are right, admirable, or good to the extent they exhibit or express benevolent motivation. (We can also assume actions are wrong or bad if they exhibit the opposite of benevolence or are somehow deficient in benevolence.) To the extent this view treats benevolence as fundamentally and inherently admirable or morally good, it is agent-based; but such a view doesn't entail that the virtuous individual with admirable inner states can simply choose any actions she pleases (among those lying within her power) without the admirability or goodness of her behavior or actions being in any way compromised or diminished. For, assuming only some reasonable form of free-will compatibilism, a benevolent agent is typically *capable* of choosing many actions that *fail to express or exhibit* her benevolence. And if one is not *entirely* or *perfectly* benevolent, then one may well be capable of choosing actions that exhibit the opposite of, or a deficiency in, this motive. Thus if one is benevolent and sees an individual who needs one's help, one may help and, in doing so, exhibit one's benevolence. But it is also presumably within one's power to refuse to help, and if one does, then one's actions won't exhibit benevolence and will presumably be less admirable than they could or would have been otherwise. Of course, the really or perfectly benevolent person will not refuse to help, but the point is that she could, and such refusal and the actions it would give rise to don't count as admirable according to the simplified agent-based view that makes benevolence the touchstone of all moral evaluation.

So it is not true to say that agent-basing entails that what one does doesn't matter morally or that it doesn't matter given that one has a good enough inner character or motivation. The person who expresses and exhibits benevolence in her actions performs actions that, in agent-based terms, can count as ethically superior to other actions she might or could have performed, namely, actions (perhaps including refrainings) that would *not* have expressed or exhibited benevolence. Acts therefore do not count as admirable or virtuous for an agent-based theory of the sort just roughly introduced merely because they are or would be done by someone who in fact is admirable or possessed of admirable motivation; acts have to exhibit, express, or further such motivation, or be such that they *would* exhibit, express, or further such motivation if they occurred, in order to qualify as admirable or virtuous. We may conclude, then, that it is simply not true that agent-based theories inevitably treat human actions as subject to no moral standards or requirements.

In order to avoid wrongdoing, one must (on agent-based theories of the sort just mentioned) avoid actions that exhibit bad or deficient inner motives (one way to do this of course would be to have perfect or univocally good inner motivation). Likewise, in order to be highly admirable, actions must express or further the realization of highly admirable inner motives. So agent-based views clearly allow for agents to be subject to moral requirements or constraints or standards governing their actions. But those requirements, standards, and constraints operate and bind, as it were, *from within*.

But even this metaphor must be taken with caution because it seems to imply that for agent-based views the direction of fit between world and moral agent is all one-way: from agent to world, and this too suggests a kind of autism or isolation from the world that makes one wonder how any such form of ethics can possibly be plausible or adequate. However, agent-basing does not entail isolation from or the irrelevance of facts about the world; in fact, the kinds of motivation such theories specify as fundamentally admirable invariably wish and need to take the world into account. If one is really benevolent, for example, one doesn't just throw good things around or give them to the first person one sees. Benevolence isn't really benevolence in the fullest sense unless one cares about who exactly is needy and to what extent they are needy, and such care, in turn, essentially involves wanting and making efforts to know relevant facts, so that one's benevolence can be really useful. Thus even if universal benevolence is a ground floor moral value, someone who acts from such a motive must be open to, seek contact with, and be influenced by the world round her – her decisions will not be made in splendid causal and epistemic isolation from what most of us would take to be the morally relevant realities, so the worries mentioned just above really have no foundation.[6]

3.   Morality as Inner Strength

Having quelled the charges of autism and antinomianism that it is initially so tempting to launch against agent-basing, I would like now to consider – too briefly, I'm afraid – how agent-based approaches might best be developed in the current climate of ethics. Looking back at the somewhat sparse history of agent-based approaches, it strikes me that there are basically two possible ways in which one may naturally develop the idea of agent-basing: one of them I call "cool," the other "warm." I mentioned earlier that Plato relates the morality of individual actions to the health and virtue of the soul, but in the *Republic* (Book IV) Plato also uses the images of a strong soul and a beautiful soul to convey what he takes to be the inner touchstone of all good human action. And I believe that ideas about health and, especially, strength can serve as the aretaic foundations for one kind of agent-based virtue ethics. Since, in addition, it is natural to wonder how any sort of *humane concern for other people* can be derived from notions like health and strength, agent-based approaches of this first kind can be conveniently classified as "cool."

By contrast, James Martineau's agent-based conception of morality treats compassion as the highest of secular motives, and some of the philosophers who have come closest to presenting agent-based views (Hume, Hutcheson, and now Jorge Garcia) have placed a special emphasis on compassion or, to use a somewhat more general term, *benevolence* as a motive. I believe the latter notion can provide the focus for a second kind of agent-based view (actually, as it turns out, a pair of views) that deserves our attention, and since this second kind of view builds humane concern explicitly into its aretaic foundations, it is natural to think of it as "warm."

Since Plato's discussion of health and strength is older than any discussion of benevolence I know, I would like first to consider agent-basing as anchored in the cool idea of strength. Metaphors of health and strength also play an important role in Stoicism, in Spinoza, and in Nietzsche, though none of these offers a perfectly clear-cut example of an agent-based account of ethics. Still, these views cluster around the same notions that fascinate and influence Plato, and I believe they can naturally be extrapolated to a modern version of Plato's virtue-ethical approach: a genuinely agent-based theory that regards inner strength, in various forms, as the sole foundation for an understanding of the morality of human action.

For Plato, good action is to be understood in terms of the seemingly consequentialistic idea of creating and/or sustaining the strength (or health, etc.) of the soul.[7] But it seems more promising to explore the idea of actions that *express* or *exhibit* inner strength, and so *morality as inner strength*, as it seems natural to call it, will proceed on that basis (without making any appeal to the supposed value of the Forms).

Now the idea that there is something intuitively admirable about being strong inside, something requiring no appeal to or defense from *other ideas*, can perhaps be made more plausible by being more specific about the kinds of inner disposition and motivation I have in mind in speaking of inner strength. What *does not* seem plausible, however, is the idea that any contemporaneously relevant and inclusive morality of human action could be based *solely* in ideas about inner strength. What does inner strength have to do with being kind to people, with not deceiving them, with not harming them? If it does not relate to these sorts of things, it clearly cannot function as a general groundwork for morality.

The same problem comes up in connection with Plato's defense of morality in the *Republic*. The *Republic* begins with the problem of explaining why anyone should be moral or just in the conventional sense of not deceiving, stealing, and the like, but Plato ends up defining justice in terms of the health or strength of the soul and never adequately explains why such a soul would refrain from what are ordinarily regarded as unjust or immoral actions. Even the appeal to the Form of the Good seems just a form of handwaving in connection with these difficulties because even though Plato holds that the healthy soul must be guided by the Good, we are not told enough about the Good to know why it would direct us away from lying and stealing. Doesn't a similar problem arise for any cool agent-based theory appealing fundamentally to the notion of inner strength? It certainly appears to, but perhaps the appearance can be dispelled by pointing out connections between certain kinds of strength and other-regarding morality that have largely gone unnoticed. Let us begin by considering how strength in the form of *self-reliance* gives rise to a concern for the well-being of others.

Most children envy the self-reliance of their parents and want to be like them, rather than continuing to depend on them or others to do things for them. Moreover, the effort to learn to do things for oneself and eventually make one's own way in the world expresses a kind of inner self-sufficiency that we think well of. The contrary desire, which we would call parasitism, is, most of us think, inherently deplorable; someone who willingly remains dependent on others rather than in any substantial degree striking out on her own seems to us pathetic and *weak*. Notice here too that the accusation of weak dependency depends more on the motivation than on the abilities of the accused. A person who is *capable* of leaving the family nest but *unwilling* to do so is considered dependent and weak and a parasite *because of his motivation*. The accusation of parasitism doesn't apply to a handicapped person who strives but fails to be entirely self-supporting or to a welfare mother in a similar position. So a morality that bases everything on *inner* strength can say that motivational (as opposed to achieved) self-reliance demonstrates inner strength and self-sufficiency and is thus inherently admirable, whereas motivational parasitism is a form of dependency and inherently weak and deplorable. It can then go on to say that acts that exhibit the one motive are right and even good, whereas those exhibiting the latter are wrong. And having appealed to our aretaic intuitions about strength and self-sufficiency in this way and without recourse to any further arguments, morality as inner strength is thus far at least an example of agent-basing. The admirability of wanting to be independent and not a parasite is not a function of its consequences for anyone's happiness, but, according to the present view, is and can be recognized to be admirable apart from any consequences. To be sure, we think it will have good results if people want to be and succeed in being self-reliant in their lives – they will help themselves and, as we shall shortly see, they will tend to help others too. (I am not assuming that attempts at *total, godlike* self-reliance make any sense for beings with our social and personal needs.) Yet our low opinion of dependent weakness is not based, or solely based, on assumptions about results.

Consider, for example, the courage it takes to face unpleasant facts about oneself or the universe. Self-deception about whether one has cancer may make the end of one's life less miserable and even make things easier for those taking care of one; but still it seems far more admirable to face such facts. Intuitively such courage is not admired for the good it does people, but rather because we find courage, and the inner or personal strength it demonstrates, inherently admirable and in need of no further defense or justification. All arguments, all theories need to start somewhere in intuitive or convincing assumptions, and in this case it would appear that the admirability of inner strength is a fundamental aretaic assumption of the sort appropriate to agent-basing.

By the same token motivational (as opposed to *achieved*) self-reliance and self-sufficiency seems admirable to us independently of any (further) argument or justification. We admire, for example, a handicapped person who makes persistent but largely unsuccessful efforts to do things for himself and earn his own money, but in such a case those efforts may frustrate and annoy the handicapped individual, and he may be less happy and contented than if he had simply allowed things to be done for him. For all we know, his motivational self-reliance might also do nothing to lift the burden of caring for him from others, and our admiration for such a person as compared with someone with no qualms about taking everything from others is thus not reasonably thought to be based on consequentialistic considerations. Rather, we seem to think of this form of strength and self-sufficiency in the same way we regard the strength to face facts, as something inherently and fundamentally admirable; and so the question now before us is: Just *how much* of our ordinary other-regarding morality can be based in considerations of inner strength?

Our admiration for self-reliance as opposed to parasitism can be used, in the first instance, to undergird and justify a good deal of activity devoted to the well-being of other people. To depend passively on society or others in the way a child depends on his parents counts as an instance of parasitism and is wrong and deplorable as such, whether we are talking about welfare chiseling, on the one hand, or, on the other, the leisured existence of the wealthy; and a person who is opposed to parasitism will presumably want to *be* useful and *make* a contribution to society, so as to counterbalance all that has been done for him by others.

Notice, furthermore, that this desire is not egoistic or self-interested, even if it presupposes one's self-interest has been served by others. For one's motive here is not the instrumental one of making a contribution in order that others may be more likely to help one in the future, but looks back to help one has already received and seeks *with no ulterior motive to counterbalance or repay that help*.

The appeal to a desire to repay and make a positive contribution to society and to particular individuals allows us to criticize both the harming of others and failures to contribute to others' well-being. But the imperative of self-reliance or non-parasitism also connects with the "deontological" side of our ordinary moral thinking – with our obligations to keep promises, not to be deceptive, to tell the truth, etc. For those who rely on others to believe their promises and who have benefitted from others' keeping promises to *them* would count as parasites upon the social practice of promising if they refused to keep their promises. More needs to be said here, but given space constraints, we ought to move on to consider some forms of inner strength we have not mentioned yet.

I have spoken of self-sufficiency understood in the sense of self-reliance, but such self-sufficiency and strength *vis-à-vis* other *people* is different from a kind of self-sufficiency in regard to *things* that we also think well of, namely, the self-sufficiency shown by those who are moderate in their needs or desires. Those who do not desire (or so strongly desire) many things that most of us desire, those who are contented with what would not be enough to satisfy most people, seem less needy, less greedy, less dependent on things than those others. Since neediness and dependency seem to be ways of being weak (inside), a certain independence from and self-sufficiency in regard to things that people can crave represents another form of inner strength that is admirable in itself.

Interestingly, this new form of self-sufficient strength can help us to justify some further kinds of altruistic behavior, and, ironically enough, it is Nietzsche, the self-avowed egoist, who shows us how to do this. The kind of moderation of desire that can be justified in terms of an ideal of self-sufficiency is not particularly directed to the good of others, but as

Nietzsche points out in *Beyond Good and Evil* (section 260), *Joyful Wisdom* (section 55), and many other places, one can also be moved to give things to other people out of a self-sufficient sense of having more than enough, a superabundance, of things. Nietzsche thinks this kind of "noble" giving is ethically superior to giving based in pity or a sense of obligation, but quite apart from this further judgment, it seems clear that Nietzsche has pointed out a further way in which benefiting others can be justified in terms of our ideal of inner strength. The person who begrudges things to others no matter how much he has seems needy, pathetic, too dependent on the things he keeps for himself, and can be criticized as lacking self-sufficiency in regard to the good things of this world.

Notice that although generosity based on this kind of self-sufficiency presupposes that the giver is genuinely satisfied with the good things she has, it is not egoistic. One generously gives to others out of a sense of one's own well-being but not in order to *promote* one's well-being or (necessarily) in order to *repay* people for previous help, and this therefore counts as a form of altruism in addition to the kind that develops out of self-reliance. Such self-sufficient generosity can serve rather widely as a touchstone for social and individual moral criticism but, once again, there is no space here to go into the details.[8] What is important at this point is that the cool notion of inner strength has sides to it that allow for a defense of various forms of altruism and of the honoring of commitments.

In fact, I believe there are four basic facets to the idea of inner strength, all with a role to play in morality as inner strength. We have mentioned three: courage to face facts and, let me add, to face danger; self-sufficient self-reliance; and self-sufficient moderation and generosity. The fourth kind of inner strength is *strength of purpose* as involving both keeping to purposes and intentions over time and following one's better judgment (not being weak-willed) at the time one is supposed to act on some intention. I don't propose at this point to go any further, though, into the details of morality as strength. Clearly, if we have four different kinds of inner strength, we need to say something about their relative importance and about how they interact to yield an intuitive and thoroughgoing account of ethical phenomena. But I want at this point to indicate a general problem with this whole approach that has led me to think there are probably more promising ways to develop an agent-based virtue ethics.

The problem, in a nutshell, is that morality as strength treats benevolence, compassion, kindness, and the like as only *derivatively* admirable and morally good; and this seems highly implausible to the modern moral consciousness. To be sure, compassion cannot always have its way; it sometimes must yield to considerations of justice, and a compassion or generosity that never pays any heed to the agent's own needs seems self-depreciating, masochistic, and ethically unattractive. But still, even if compassion has to be limited or qualified by other values, it counts with us as a *very important basic moral value*. And it seems to distort the aretaic value we place on warm compassion, benevolence, and kindness to regard them as needing justification in terms of the cool ideal of inner strength or any other different value. (Such a criticism clearly also touches the Kantian account of benevolence.) So I would propose at this point to introduce and discuss certain warm forms of agent-based virtue ethics that are immune to this problem precisely because they base all morality on the aretaic value, the moral admirability, of one or another kind of benevolence. Moreover, as I mentioned earlier, Martineau's *Types of Ethical Theory* is the clearest example of agent-basing one can find in the entire history of ethics, and I believe that the advantages of virtue ethics based on compassion or benevolence can best be brought to light by first considering the structure of Martineau's theory and the criticisms that Henry Sidgwick made of that theory.

4. Morality as Universal Benevolence

Martineau gives a ranking of human motives from lowest to highest and, assuming that all moral decisions involve a conflict between two such motives, holds that right action is action from the higher of the two motives, and wrong action action from the lower of the two.[9] Martineau's hierarchy of motives ascends (roughly) as follows: vindictiveness; love of sensual pleasure; love of gain; resentment–fear–antipathy; ambition–love of power; compassion; and, at the apex, reverence for the Deity.

Sidgwick objects to the rigidity of this hierarchy, pointing out that circumstances and consequences may affect the preferability of acting from one or another of the motives Martineau has ranked.[10] Thus contrary to Martineau, there are times when it is better for reasons of justice to act from resentment rather than compassion, and the love of sensual pleasure might sometimes prevail over a love of power or gain (especially if the latter were already being given ample play). Sidgwick concludes that conflicts between lower motives can only be resolved by appeal to the highest ranked motive or, alternatively, to some supremely regulative general motive like justice, prudence, or universal benevolence – none of which is contained among the more particular motives of Martineau's hierarchy. That is, all conflicts of Martineau's lower motives should be settled by reference to reverence for the Deity or by reference to some regulative or "master" motive like benevolence. (This would not be necessary if we could devise a more plausible and less priggish hierarchy than Martineau's, but no one has yet suggested a way of doing that.)

Sidgwick then goes on to make one further mistake, assumption. He assumes that for a motive to be regulative, it must be regulative in relation to the ultimate *ends* or *goals* of that motive. This entails that if we confine ourselves to secular motives, take seriously the fact that compassion is the highest secular motive in Martineau's ranking, and as a result choose universal benevolence as supremely regulative, then actions and motives will be judged in terms of the goal of universal benevolence, namely, human or sentient happiness. Somehow, we have ended up not with a more orderly or unified form of agent-based view, but with *act-utilitarianism*. And this has happened because Sidgwick ignores the possibility of an agent-based view that judges actions from either of two conflicting motives in terms of how well the two motives exemplify or approximate to the motive of universal benevolence, *rather than* in terms of whether those actions achieve (or are likely to achieve) certain goals that universal benevolence aims at.

Thus suppose someone knows that he can help a friend in need, but that he could instead have fun swimming. The good he can do for himself by swimming is a great deal less than what he can do for his friend, but he also knows that if he swims, certain strangers will somehow indirectly benefit and the benefit will be greater than anything he can provide for his needy friend. However the man doesn't at all care about the strangers, and though he does care about his friend, he ends up taking a swim. In that case, both actualist and expectabilist versions of act-utilitarianism will regard his action as the morally best available to him in the circumstances. It has better consequences for human happiness than any alternative, and its expectable utility is greater than the alternative of helping his friend, since the man *knows* he will do more good, directly and indirectly, by swimming. But there is a difference between *expecting* or *knowing* that an act will have good consequences and *being motivated* to produce those consequences, and if we judge actions in agent-based fashion by how closely their motives exemplify or approximate to universal benevolence, then it is morally *less* good for him to go swimming for his selfish reason than to try to help his needy friend, and this is precisely the opposite of what standard forms of act-utilitarianism would conclude.

Thus in order to rule out agent-based views making use of the notion of compassion or benevolence, it is not enough to undermine complicated views like Martineau's, for we have seen that there can be an agent-based *analogue* (or *"interiorization"*) of utilitarianism that morally judges everything, in unified or monistic fashion, by reference to universal benevolence as a *motive that seeks* certain ends rather than, in the utilitarian manner, by reference to the actual or probable *occurrence* of those ends. In addition, this distinctive *morality as universal benevolence* contrasts with utilitarianism in some striking further ways we have not yet mentioned.

Utilitarians and other consequentialists evaluate motives and intentions in the same way as actions, namely, in terms of their consequences. (I shall here ignore rule-utilitarianism because of what I take to be its inherent difficulties.) Thus consider someone whose motives would ordinarily be thought not to be morally good, a person who gives money for the building of a hospital, but who is motivated only by a desire to see her name on a building or a desire to get a reputation for generosity as a means to launching a political career. Utilitarians and consequentialists will typically say that her particular motivation, her motivation in those circumstances, is morally good, whereas morality as universal benevolence, because it evaluates motives in terms of how well they approximate to universal benevolence, will be able, more intuitively, to treat such motivation as less than morally good (even if not very *bad* either). Of course, when we learn of what such a person is doing and of her selfish motivation, we may well be happy and think it a good thing that she has the egotistical motives she has on the occasion in question, given their good consequences (and our own benevolence). But we ordinarily distinguish between motives that, relative to circumstances we are glad to see and it is good to have occur and those motives we genuinely admire as morally good. Consequentialism, however, standardly leads to a denial and collapse of this plausible distinction by morally evaluating motives solely in terms of their consequences. By contrast, morality as universal benevolence, precisely because it insists that the *moral* evaluation of motives depends on their inherent character as motives rather than on their consequences, allows for the distinction and comes much closer to an intuitive conception of what makes motives morally better or worse.

As an agent-based analogue of utilitarianism, morality as universal benevolence is, however, open to many of the criticisms that have recently been directed at utilitarianism, including the claim that such views demand too much self-sacrifice. But this last problem can perhaps be dealt with on analogy with the way utilitarianism and consequentialism have attempted to deal with the criticism of overdemandingness: namely, either by arguing against it outright, or by accommodating it through an adjustment of their principle(s) of right action. A satisficing version of (utilitarian) consequentialism can say that right action requires only that one do *enough* good, and it can then offer some agent-neutral conception of what it is, in various situations, to do enough good for humankind considered as a whole. And a satisficing version of morality as universal benevolence can say (in a manner indicated above) that acts are right if they come from a motive (together with underlying moral dispositions) that is *close enough* to universal benevolence – rather than insisting that only acts exemplifying the highest motive, universal benevolence, can count as morally acceptable. Someone who devoted most of her time, say, to the rights of consumers or to peace in Northern Ireland might then count as acting and living rightly, even if she were not concerned with universal human welfare and sometimes preferred simply to enjoy herself. So there are versions of morality as universal benevolence that allow us to meet the criticism of overdemandingness, even if we think that this criticism does have force against versions of the view that require us always to have the morally best motives or moral dispositions when we act.

Some forms of utilitarianism are also, however, criticized for having an overly narrow conception of human well-being and in particular for treating all well-being as a matter of the balance of pleasure over pain. This criticism doesn't hold for certain pluralistic forms of consequentialism, nor does it apply to morality as universal benevolence, interestingly enough. The latter is not committed to any particular conception of human well-being, and happily allows us to admire a person's concern and compassion for human beings without attributing to that person or ourselves having a settled view of what human well-being consists in.

Finally, utilitarianism has been criticized for its inability to account for certain aspects of deontology, and these criticisms would undoubtedly also extend to morality as universal benevolence. Strict deontology tells us we would be wrong to kill one person in a group in order to prevent everyone in the group, including the person in question, from being killed by some menacing third party. But although Kantian ethics indeed seems to demand that we refrain from killing the one person, it is not clear that our ordinary thinking actually insists on such a requirement. Bernard Williams, for example, says that the question whether to kill one to save the rest is more difficult than utilitarianism can allow, but he also grants that utilitarianism probably gives the right answer about what to do in such a case.[11] Moreover, since benevolence involves not only the desire to do what is good or best overall for the people one is concerned about, *but also the desire that no one of those people should suffer*, morality as universal benevolence can explain why we might be horrified at killing one to save many, even if in the end it holds that that is what we morally ought to do.

I conclude, then, that although both consequentialism and morality as universal benevolence are open to a good many familiar criticisms, they have ways of responding to the criticisms. Moreover, they have systematic advantages over many other approaches to morality because of their relative systematicity or unified structure. But, as I suggested earlier, morality as universal benevolence seems to have intuitive advantages over its more familiar utilitarian/consequentialist analogues. Though it is a view that to the best of my knowledge has not previously been explicitly stated or defended, it is in many ways more commonsensical and plausible than utilitarianism and consequentialism. At the same time its reliance on the ideas of benevolence and universality should render it attractive to defenders of the latter views and make them ask themselves whether it wouldn't be better to accept an agent-based "interiorized" version of their own doctrines. If consequentialism and utilitarianism have present-day viability and appeal, agent-based morality as universal benevolence does too.[12]

5. Morality as Caring

We have not yet exhausted the promising possibilities of agent-basing, and at this point I would like to consider one final way of utilizing the idea of benevolence within an agent-based virtue ethics. Some educationists and philosophers have recently been exploring and developing the idea of an ethic or morality of *caring*, and I would like now to push or disambiguate this idea in the direction of a new kind of warm agent-based view.

It is possible to ground an agent-based ethical theory in an ideal of *partial or particularistic benevolence*, of caring *more* for some than for others. We find at least the potential for such a view in St. Augustine's claim that all virtue is based in love for God (though at various points Augustine appears to import non-agent-based elements into his arguments).[13] But it is also possible to develop a purely secular agent-based view that puts a premium on caring for or benevolence toward some people more than others, and it is this possibility that I want to consider in what follows.

In her ground-breaking *In a Different Voice*, Carol Gilligan argued that men tend to conceive morality in terms of rights, justice, and autonomy, whereas women more frequently think of the moral in terms of caring, responsibility, and interrelation with others. At about the same time Nel Noddings, in *Caring: A Feminine Approach to Ethics and Moral Education*, sought to articulate and defend in its own right a "feminine" morality centered specifically around the idea of caring.[14] But when one reads Noddings, one is left unclear as to whether she intends her ethics of caring to be agent-based. The notion of agent-basing has only recently become a tool of ethical theory, and there is no reason to expect Noddings, writing some years back, to have related her work to that notion. But given recent developments, especially in virtue ethics, it is perhaps interesting to consider whether the morality of caring cannot be seen as agent-based and thereby given a firmer or more definite theoretical grounding.

In her book, Noddings seems to want to relate everything in morality to particularistic caring, rather than bringing in independent principles of justice or truth-telling or what-have-you, but there is still a potential obstacle to seeing her ethics as agent-based. For although she emphasizes the moral goodness of acting from care, she also says that we should try to *promote* caring in the world, and this sounds like a consequentialistic and indeed perfectionistic element in her views. (Perfectionism is a form of consequentialism that tells us, roughly, to focus ultimately on whether our acts produce virtue and excellence, not on their results for happiness.) If she believes in a fundamental imperative to produce or promote caring in the world, then Noddings's view is clearly not agent-based, but I don't think what we know of Noddings's views settles the issue because she never says that the promotion of caring is a fundamental moral value, and if it is not, then there is in fact a way of *deriving* it from an agent-based partialistic ethic of caring.

Consider the reasons one might have for trying to get (certain) people to care more about (certain other) people. Couldn't one's reason be that by getting them to care more, one could eventually bring about more good for humanity generally or for the people one cares about? If one really wants to help (certain) people, working to get them to care for one another's welfare might have a multiplier effect, allowing one at least indirectly to help more people overall than if one always simply promoted welfare directly. A caring person might thus see the promotion of caring as the best way to promote what she as a caring person is concerned about. In that measure, the concern for and promotion of virtuous caring on the part of others would be an instance of caring itself conceived as a fundamental form of moral excellence, and would thus be accommodatable within an agent-based theory of the moral value of caring. Perfectionism and good results as such would not have to come into the matter. But as I say, I am not sure Noddings is best interpreted in this way and only suggest it because the agent-based theory we have just arrived at is, at the very least, interesting and promising in its own right.

An agent-based moral theory that puts a moral premium on particularistic caring presumably needs to say more than Noddings says about self-concern and about appropriate attitudes and actions toward strangers. No reasonable ethics should decry or begrudge self-concern and a degree of self-assertiveness in moral agents. As feminists and others have recently noted, it would be ironic and morally counter-productive for any new ethics to focus exclusively on aspects of feminine moral thought and activity that have typically restricted women. An ethic of care primarily for favored *others* seems, then, to be morally retrograde; but there is no reason why a specifically agent-based feminine or feminist ethic of caring shouldn't say that it is best to be motivated by concern for others *in balance with* self-concern, and that all and only actions that are consonant with and display such balance are morally acceptable.[15]

There is also the problem of appropriate concern for and treatment of strangers. But a partialistic morality that advocated greater concern for near and dear might still deplore *indifference* to strangers, and if the moral floor of non-indifference, of humane caring, is not set too low, an agent-based morality as caring will be able to treat the usual questions of justice and human rights in a plausible, but highly distinctive way.[16]

Defenders of universality and impartiality may object at this point that the ethic of caring does not provide *enough* assurance that strangers will be properly treated and so argue for the theoretical preferability of morality as universal benevolence among agent-based doctrines. But partialists can reply that devotion to particular individuals seems morally preferable to and more admirable than any sort of impartial benevolence, and it is not clear who has the better case here. Note however that some partialists claim that particularistic caring is obligatory and admirable because it is *necessary to important human goods* that are realizable only in close relationships. Such an explanation takes us away from agent-basing, but I wonder how cogent it is. If parental love is obligatory and admirable *because* essential to the good(s) of family life, why isn't a child just as obligated to take things from her parents and accounted admirable for doing so? The difference here seems to depend on a *fundamental difference in admirability* between caring for and being cared for, and that sits well with an agent-based morality that deems caring admirable as such and apart from its helping to realize certain goods. Similarly, the devotion of a tutor to a mentally handicapped child can be very admirable, even if it might be *better* if their relationship weren't needed. The admirability of such caring seems not to be grounded in the desirability of a relationship, but, again, to stand in no need of further justification; so a morality of caring should have no qualms, I think, about conceiving of itself as agent-based.

6. Can Agent-Based Theories be Applied?

However, our two favored forms of agent-based virtue ethics – morality as universal benevolence and morality as caring – face a further difficulty that must now be mentioned. If someone is faced with a perplexing moral problem, it somehow seems irrelevant and even objectionable for her to examine *her own motives rather than facts about people and the world* in order to solve it. Yet isn't this what agent-basing allows for and even prescribes? Doesn't, for example, morality as (universal or partialistic) benevolence tell us that whether it is morally good, right, or acceptable, say, to oppose the taking of heroic measures to keep an aged dying parent alive depends on the motives of the person in question? And is this at all helpful for someone who *doesn't know* whether to advocate or oppose heroic measures for a dying or suffering parent? Looking inward at or for motives presumably won't help to solve that person's problem, and so where we most need moral guidance, it would seem that agent-basing not only is irrelevant but makes it impossible to find a solution to one's moral difficulties.

Some defenders of virtue ethics are willing to grant that virtue ethics – whether agent-based or otherwise – cannot be applied to practical moral issues, but would claim nonetheless that virtue ethics can give us the correct theory or view of morality.[17] However, it would be better for virtue ethics if we could show that (agent-based) virtue ethics *can* be applied, and I believe we can accomplish this by making further use of the way that an internal state like benevolence focuses on and concerns itself with gathering facts about the world. If one morally judges a certain course of action or decision by reference to, say, the benevolence of the motives of its agent, one is judging in relation to an inner factor that itself takes into account facts about people in the world. One's inward gaze effectively "doubles back" on the world and allows one, as we shall see in more detail in a moment, to take facts about the world into account in one's attempt to determine what is morally acceptable or best to do. On the other hand this doubling back is not unnecessarily duplicative or wasteful of moral effort, if we assume that motive is fundamentally at least relevant to the *moral* character of any action. For if we judge the actions of ourselves or others simply by their effects in the world, we end up unable to distinguish accidentally or ironically useful actions (or slips on banana peels) from actions that we actually morally admire and that are morally good and praiseworthy.

Consider, then, someone who hears that her aged mother has suddenly been taken to the hospital and who flies from a distant city to be with her. Given morality as benevolence in some form or other and assuming she is her mother's sole living relative, how should she resolve the issue of what morally she ought to do with or for her parent when she gets to the hospital: Should she or should she not, for example, advocate heroic measures to save her mother? Surely morality as some form of benevolence doesn't give her an answer to this question, but what is worth noting is that given the woman's assumed ignorance of her mother's particular condition and prospects, there is no reason for most moral theories to offer an answer to that question at this point. But morality as benevolence *does* offer her an answer to the question what morally she should do when she gets to the hospital. It tells her she morally ought (would be wrong not) to find out more about her mother's condition and prospects, as regards quality and duration of life and certainly as regards future suffering and incapacity. And it can tell her this by reference to her actual motives, because if she does not find out more and decides what to do or to advocate about her mother solely on the basis of present relative ignorance, she will demonstrate a callousness (toward her mother) that is very far from benevolent. To decide to pull the plug or not allow heroic measures without finding out more about her mother would demonstrate indifference or callousness toward her and on that basis morality as benevolence can make the moral judgment that she ought to find out more before making any decision. (Morality as inner strength could be shown to yield a similar conclusion.)

Then, once the facts have emerged, and assuming they are fairly clear-cut and point to horrendously painful and debilitating prospects for her mother, the woman's decision is once again plausibly derivable from morality as benevolence. At that point, it would be callous of her to insist on heroic measures and benevolent not to do so, and the proper moral decision can thus be reached by agent-based considerations.

But surely, someone might say, the woman herself does not think in such terms. She is worried about whether her mother would have a painful or pleasant future existence, for example, not about whether she herself would be acting callously if she sought to prolong the mother's existence. I would think that she could morally justify her decision not to allow heroic measures *either* by reference simply to likely future suffering if the mother were kept alive, or by saying, more complexly and richly: it would be (would have been) callous of me to try to keep her alive, given her prospects. Surely, there is nothing unusual or untoward about the latter as an expression of moral problem-solving.[18]

Think, for example, about the arguments that were made in advocacy of the North American Free Trade Agreement (NAFTA). Both Vice President Gore and House Minority Leader Robert Michel defended the agreement on the grounds that to reject it would be to adopt a cringing, fearful, or despairing attitude to the world and America's future. They could have spoken more directly about consequences, but there is nothing unreasonable about the way they addressed the issue. So I want to conclude that, given the outward-looking character of inner motives, agent-based views have resources for the resolution of moral issues that parallel those available to such practically applicable moral theories as utilitarianism and consequentialism more generally.

Our ordinary thinking in response to difficult or not-so-difficult practical moral issues can invoke either motives or consequences or both. Consequentialism, however, solves such issues by appealing ultimately to consequences and only indirectly and as a method of useful approximation to considerations of motives like impartial benevolence. Agent-based morality as benevolence solves the problem in the opposite fashion by appealing ultimately to motives, but taking in consequences indirectly, to the extent they are considered by people with such motives and investigated in response to such motives. Each approach allows for the case-by-case solution of many moral difficulties or problems, and so with regard to the whole question of applied ethics, neither approach seems to have the advantage, and there is no reason to criticize agent-basing for being irrelevant to practical moral problems or making their solutions impossible.[19]

To be sure, there will be times when morality as benevolence won't be able to solve our moral difficulties. For example, if the facts about her mother's prospects cannot be learned or turn out to be highly complicated, morality as benevolence will be stymied. But any consequentialism worthy of the name will also come up empty in such a case. It is a strength of such views, but no less of agent-based morality as benevolence, whether in partialistic or universalistic form, that such views do not presume to know the answers to difficult moral questions in cases that *outrun our human knowledge or reasoning powers*. Any ethical theory that makes it too easy always to know what to do or to feel will seem to that extent flawed or even useless because untrue to our soberer sense of the wrenching complexity of moral phenomena.

Since the revival of virtue ethics, those interested in the subject have focused mainly on Aristotle and on neo-Aristotelian ideas. I have myself defended neo-Aristotelian agent-focused ideas *From Morality to Virtue*, but we have seen here that certain forms of agent-based virtue ethics also have real promise and possibilities. In a period when virtue ethics is flexing its muscles, it needs a more varied diet than Aristotle or Aristotelianism alone can provide.

Notes

1 For a discussion of what it is for an ethical view to count as a form of virtue ethics, see my *From Morality to Virtue* (Oxford, 1992), Chapter 5, and Marcia Baron's "Varieties of Ethics of Virtue," *American Philosophical Quarterly* 22 (1985), 52n. I shall not much stress the fact that virtue theories are supposed to prefer aretaic characterizations in terms of excellence, moral goodness, or admirability to deontic evaluations making use of notions like "ought," "wrong," and "obligation."

2 In "Virtue Theory and Abortion" (*Philosophy and Public Affairs* 20 [1991]: 223–46), Rosalind Hursthouse interprets Aristotle as deriving all evaluations of actions from independent judgments about what counts as a virtue, but basing the latter, in turn, in judgments about, a conception of, *eudaimonia*. But if Aristotle regards virtuous living as the primary component of *eudaimonia*, it becomes difficult to see how Aristotelianism can be grounded in the way indicated by Hursthouse. In any event, such an interpretation doesn't treat Aristotelian ethics as agent-based: act-evaluations may be derivative from independent aretaic character evaluations, but the latter are not fundamental and are supposed to be grounded in a theory or view of *eudaimonia*. (I assume here that *eudaimonia* and the ideas of well-being and a good life are not themselves aretaic, even though some ethical views treat them as closely connected to or based in aretaic notions. On this point see my *From Morality to Virtue*, Chapter 13.)

3 Ideal observer theories (and response dependence views) are not necessarily agent-based, for even if they define rightness in terms of the attitudes of an observer defined as having what are ordinarily considered to be virtues, e.g., disinterestedness, objectivity, or lack of bias, the theory doesn't (needn't) *say* that these inner traits are virtues or attempt to spell out what all the virtues are independently of its specification of the right. Indeed, on standard formulations, ideal observer theories leave it open that an ideal observer should condemn her own disinterestedness or lack of bias, and so such theories clearly do not commit themselves to any account of good inner traits or motives as the basis for their accounts of right action.

4 Sidgwick, *Methods of Ethics*, seventh edition (London, 1967), 202.

5   Similar worries could also occur about views (like Aristotle as interpreted by Hursthouse) that treat act-evaluations as derivative from aretaic agent-characterizations but base the latter in some other type of ethical consideration. The worries are misplaced for exactly the same reasons described in the main text in connection with agent-basing.

6   Of course, if someone makes every effort to learn about things and is foiled by reality or his own innate lack of intelligence, his benevolence will not have its intended effect and may actually cause a great deal of harm. But the personal defect here, if any, is presumably cognitive, not moral. So when such an agent brings about bad results, an agent-based view may still plausibly say that the agent didn't act morally wrongly. (Even then we might say that the agent didn't "do the right thing"; but that is a more objective use of 'right' and is not the act-characterizing moral notion agent-based virtue ethics *primarily* wishes to capture.)

7   Plato, *Republic*, Book IV, S. 443–4.

8   For more on how the motive of self-sufficient generosity tends to limit individual acquisitiveness and to lead toward social egalitarianism, see my "Virtue Ethics and Democratic Values," *Journal of Social Philosophy* 24 (1993), 5–37.

9   See Martineau, *Types of Ethical Theory*, 2 volumes (Oxford, 1891).

10   See Sidgwick, *Methods of Ethics*, Book 3, Chapter 7.

11   See his "A Critique of Utilitarianism," in J. Smart and B. Williams, *Utilitarianism: For and Against* (Cambridge, 1985), esp. 117.

12   In his *Inquiry into the Original of Our Idea of Virtue* (excerpted in this volume), Francis Hutcheson takes universal benevolence to be inherently the morally best or highest motive, but evaluates actions in terms of how well they further the goal(s) of such benevolence. Such a view lies midway between morality as universal benevolence and utilitarianism, morally assessing motives in the manner of the former, but actions in the manner of the latter. As a result it is open to the usual objections that are made of hybrid moral views (like rule-utilitarianism).

13   Augustine, *De Moribus Ecclesiae Catholicae*, 15.25.

14   See Carol Gilligan, *In a Different Voice: Psychological Theory and Women's Development* (Cambridge, Mass., 1982); and Nel Noddings, *Caring: A Feminine Approach to Ethics and Moral Education* (Berkeley and Los Angeles, 1984).

15   On the idea that we should balance self-concern with concern for other people (considered as a class), see my *From Morality to Virtue*, Chapter 6. However I am not denying that it is often difficult to disentangle self-interest from altruism, as, for example, when the help one has given one's own children or a friend represents a happy achievement of one's own life.

16   In a 1988 talk to the Society for Women in Philosophy, Noddings said that our obligations to strangers cannot be accommodated through the notion of caring, because caring requires an ongoing relationship. But rather than give up on the idea of a total morality of caring in this way, I think we should try

to make sense of the idea of a morally requisite minimum level of concern for distant strangers (who after all do share the planet and many other things with us). Virginia Held in *Feminist Morality* (Chicago, 1993, 223) makes some suggestive remarks in this direction.

17   See, for example, Edmund Pincoffs, *Quandaries and Virtues* (St. Lawrence, Kansas, 1986).

18   If the woman thinks "I mustn't keep her alive, because if I do, I won't deserve to be considered – or be able to regard myself as – a kind person," she is self-absorbed and shows herself less than ideally benevolent or kind. But the mere thought that it would be unkind or callous if one were to keep one's mother alive, given her prospects, seems compatible with the highest kindness. The reference to one's own motives required for the practical application of an agent-based morality as benevolence need in no way undercut the benevolence that such a view prizes.

19   I am not assuming that someone who is benevolent or accepts a theory like morality as (universal or partial) benevolence has to think explicitly in moral terms to find the answer to a practical moral question. If she just wants to know what would be the (most) benevolent thing to do, finds out, and then acts accordingly, we may well want to regard her as thereby having answered the practical moral question others might pose using explicitly moral language. But that is not to say that such a person *cannot* deal with moral difficulties in explicitly moral terms. A benevolent person can easily be concerned to do what is right *given her own view that benevolence defines or determines rightness.*

Part III

Contemporary Discussion

10

On the Primacy of Character

Gary Watson

1

John Rawls taught us to think of moral theory as treating primarily three concepts: the concept of right (wrong, permissible), the concept of good, and the concept of moral worth. Of these concepts, however, he takes the latter to be derivative: "The two main concepts of ethics are those of the right and the good; the concept of a morally worthy person is, I believe, derived from them. The structure of an ethical theory is, then, largely determined by how it defines and connects these two basic notions."[1] Thus Rawls recognizes two types of theories: those that "define" the right in terms of the good and those that do not. Rawls's own theory illustrates the second type. An example of the first is classical utilitarianism, which "defines" right action as maximizing human happiness (or the satisfaction of rational desire), which is taken to be the intrinsic or ultimate good.

On either of the types of theory that Rawls recognizes, the concept of moral worth (which includes that of virtue) will be subordinated to one of the other concepts. For example, on Rawls's theory (as well as on broadly Kantian theories generally), virtues are construed as "strong and normally effective desires to act on the basic principles of right" (1971, p. 436). Some versions of utilitarianism may accept this construal as well, or else define virtues directly in terms of the good that certain traits or dispositions will do.

Gary Watson, "On the Primacy of Character," *Identity, Character, and Morality*, edited by Owen Flanagan and Amelie Rorty (Cambridge, MA: MIT Press, 1990), pp. 449–69.

Recently a number of philosophers have expressed dissatisfaction with this kind of scheme on the grounds that it precludes from the outset views that give to virtue a more central place (such as those by and large of the ancients). My aim is to investigate whether or not this dissatisfaction is well grounded. The alleged alternative has not, in my opinion, been sufficiently, or even roughly, articulated. I wish, then, to explore the structure of "ethics of virtue," as they are usually called, to determine whether they indeed constitute theories of a third kind.

2

Rawls's twofold scheme corresponds to another prevalent division of theories into "teleological" and "deontological." These theories are ways of relating the two concepts that Rawls takes to be basic. In teleological views "the good is defined independently from the right, and then the right is defined as that which maximizes the good" (1971, p. 24).[2] Teleological theories are, in a word, consequentialist. The contrasting conception is defined negatively as what is not teleological. As a result, all moral theories are construed as either consequentialist or deontological.

The awkwardness of this taxonomy can be seen by applying it to the case of Aristotle. Rawls considers Aristotle a teleologist (of the perfectionist variety). This classification would have us think of Aristotle's view as differing from utilitarianism only in its conception of what is to be maximized. But that is very doubtful. For Aristotle, the virtuous person is not one who is out to maximize anything, nor is virtue itself defined as a state that tends to promote some independently definable good (these being the two ways in which virtue can be treated in a broadly consequentialist theory).

So Aristotle's theory is deontological if that just means nonconsequentialist. But this classification seems equally inapt.[3] For a concept of good *is* primary in Aristotle's view. Thus if teleological theories are those in which the (or a) concept of the good is primary, then Aristotle's theory is rightly said to be teleological. It is a mistake, however, to think that the only way of asserting the primacy of the good is consequentialism. We should recognize the possibility of a view that is at once teleological and nonconsequentialist. An ethics of virtue, I shall suggest, is a theory of this kind.[4]

We can avoid some unfortunate conflations by replacing this distinction as Rawls draws it with the threefold distinction that his discussion originally suggests: an ethics of requirement, an ethics of consequences, and an ethics of virtue or character. This classification enables us to observe that while both ethics of consequences and ethics of virtue are teleological insofar as they are guided fundamentally by a notion of the good, Aristotle is nonetheless closer to Kant than to Bentham on the question of consequentialism. It also enables us to consider what it means to take the concept of virtue as fundamental.

3

Before I go on to consider this question more fully, I should note that the phrase "ethics of virtue" is often used in a different way from the way in which it will be used here. Some writers use this phrase to indicate something to live by (Frankena 1970), a certain moral outlook that calls for exclusive moral attention to questions about character and the quality of one's whole life. The contrast here is supposed to be with an "ethics of duty or principle," in which the fundamental moral questions are about what one's duty is and how to do it.

This is not at all the contrast that concerns me in this chapter. In the sense that concerns me, an ethics of virtue is not a code or a general moral claim but a set of abstract theses about how certain concepts are best fitted together for the purposes of understanding morality. To claim that we should give exclusive moral attention either to questions of duty or to questions of character seems to me a very special and suspect position. A morally admirable person will, for example, acknowledge her duties as a teacher to read her students' work carefully and promptly, acknowledge her obligation to repay a loan, and acknowledge the principle never to take bribes as a juror. No doubt we will disagree in some cases about what duties there are and what they involve (whether a democratic citizen has a duty to vote, for instance) and about the importance of certain duties relative to one another and to other considerations. Nonetheless, to say that questions of duty or principle never take moral precedence (or always do) seems morally incorrect.

To think that an ethics of virtue in my sense is opposed to duty is a category mistake. Duties and obligations are simply factors to which certain values, for example, fidelity and justice, are responsive. They do not compete with virtue for moral attention.

4

While it might have implications for how one lives, an ethics of virtue is not, like an ethics of love or liberation, a moral outlook or ideal but a claim that the concept of virtue is in some way theoretically dominant. On an ethics of virtue, how it is best or right or proper to conduct oneself is explained in terms of how it is best for a human being to be. I will call this the *claim of explanatory primacy*.

Explanatory primacy can be realized in different ways by different theories. One straightforward way, for example, is to explain right conduct as what accords with the virtues.[5] To be explanatory, of course, virtue must be intelligible independently of the notion of right conduct. That requirement would be violated by the Rawlsian definition of the virtues as attachments to the principles of right.

But I have formulated the thesis too narrowly, for it should also encompass terms of appraisal besides "right." It should include more generally the concepts that fall under the heading of "morally good conduct." An ethics of virtue is not a particular claim about the priority of virtue over right conduct but the more general claim that action appraisal is derivative from the appraisal of character. To put it another way, the claim is that the basic moral facts are facts about the quality of character. Moral facts about action are ancillary to these.

Indeed, some recent writers have been deeply distrustful of the general notions of moral right and wrong; they question whether there *are* any facts about right and wrong of the kind that moral philosophers want to explain. They recommend the *replacement* of talk about moral right and wrong with talk about the virtues. As G. E. M. Anscombe puts it, "It would be a great improvement if, instead of 'morally wrong,' one always named a genus such as 'untruthful,' 'unchaste,' 'unjust.' We should no longer ask whether doing something was 'wrong,' passing directly from some description of an action to this notion; we should ask whether, e.g., it was unjust; and the answer would sometimes be clear at once."[6]

I shall extend the interpretation of the thesis of explanatory priority to accommodate replacement views. This is admittedly a stretch, since on the most radical view, virtue concepts achieve priority by default. (Unless otherwise noted, when I speak of the claim of explanatory primacy hereafter I mean to include both the reductionist and the replacement interpretations.)

5

If "right" and "wrong" are contrary predicates, then the thesis of explanatory primacy commits ethics of virtue (in their nonreplacement versions) to a kind of harmony among the virtues. If it were possible for someone to act in accordance with one virtue while acting contrary to another, one's conduct would in that case be both right and wrong. This implication can be avoided if no virtue can be exercised in a way that is contrary to another. In this way, ethics of virtue is naturally led to embrace a historically controversial thesis.[7]

The controversy is avoided altogether by rejecting the idea that "right" and "wrong" are contraries. It might also be avoided by a sufficiently radical replacement view. The view would have to replace not only "right" and "wrong" but also "proper" and "improper," "licit" and "illicit," for these too seem to be contraries.

6

Another tenet often associated with ethics of virtue is uncodifiability, that is, that there are no formulas that can serve as exact and detailed guides for action. Aristotle expresses this idea in the following passage: "How far and how much we must deviate to be blamed is not easy to define in an account; for nothing perceptible is easily defined, and [since] these [circumstances of virtuous and vicious actions] are particulars, the judgment about them depends on perception" (*Nicomachean Ethics* 1109a21f). I shall confine myself to three general remarks on this idea.

First, this thesis is difficult to evaluate because codifiability seems to be a matter of degree. On the one hand, there are true moral generalizations about conduct, as even the proponents of uncodifiability should agree; on the other hand, the most rigid codifiers should concede that judgment is necessary for interpreting and applying any rules and principles. The uncodifiability thesis is supposed to be opposed to classical utilitarian and Kantian formulas, although these are far from exact and detailed. So it is unclear what counts as too much codification.

In the second place, uncodifiability is not strictly a corollary of an ethics of virtue. It is not incompatible with explanatory primacy to suppose that right action could be determined according to a clear and definite general criterion. If it could be shown that some principle of right action could somehow be derived from and explained by the conditions for being a virtuous human being, then the resulting view would still deserve to be called an ethics of virtue. Such a derivation would be perfectly consistent with the claim of explanatory primacy. Right action is acting in accordance with the virtues, but it might turn out that some principle(s), even the principle of utility or the categorical imperative, characterizes what the virtues would lead a person to do.

In this connection, it is sometimes said that in an ethics of principles or duties, it is the principles or duties that tell you what to do, whereas in an ethics of virtue, it is virtue that tells you what to do. So it might be supposed that if such principles were available (if morality were codifiable), virtue would lose this distinctive role. This thought seems to me to be somewhat confused. In the sense in which a principle can tell one what to do, namely by expressing or implying a prescriptive conclusion about action, a virtue cannot tell anything. A virtue is not a proposition one can consult or apply or interpret; it does not in the same sense prescribe any course of action. Only something like a principle can do that. On the other hand, one's virtues may enable one to endorse, apprehend, correctly apply, or disregard some principle of action. But they will also have this role in an ethics of consequences or requirement. The principle of utility may tell agents what to do, but it is their virtue that leads them to listen, interpret, and to follow.

I conclude that the uncodifiability thesis is not something to which every version of an ethics of virtue is committed. Nonetheless (and this is my third point), the relation between uncodifiability and ethics of virtue is not merely an accidental association. One of the main impetuses for the recent resurgence of interest in ethics of virtue, I suspect, is the sense that the enterprise of articulating principles of right has failed. On the Rawlsian view, that failure leaves the concept of virtue (as attachment to the right) altogether at sea. The content of virtue, if it has any, would have to come from somewhere else. One of the appeals of ethics of virtue, I conjecture, is that it promises a nonskeptical response to the failure of codification.

7

An alternative response to the failure of codification is traditional intuitionism. We have just seen that uncodifiability is not necessarily a tenet of an ethics of virtue. Since that thesis is compatible with the right being prior to the good, it is even more clearly not sufficient for an ethics of virtue. Some intuitionists may think of virtue(s) as attachment(s) to right conduct, as intuitively apprehended in particular circumstances, or perhaps better as capacities for discernment and commitment to right conduct. More generally, if intuitionism is defined as any nonskeptical view of right conduct that rejects codifiability, then some ethics of virtue are species of intuitionism.[8] More familiar members of the genus would be distinguished by their acceptance of a different direction of priority between the concepts of right and virtue.

Because of the preferred direction of priority of an ethics of virtue, its theoretical power clearly depends upon its theory of virtue. Once more, the concept of proper or right conduct will be well understood only if the concept of virtue is. Though some will hold that we can understand what the virtues are and how they are expressed without the benefit of any general theory,[9] the thesis of explanatory primacy will then be quite gratuitous. If the alleged priority cannot be established by an account, in this case a theory of virtue, then the distinction between virtue intuitionism and act intuitionism seems merely to be nominal. I question whether "prior" has any sense here whatever.

To be interesting and, I suspect, even to be meaningful, the priority claim has to occur as part of a theory of virtue. I shall take it, then, that an ethics of virtue will have two components:

a. Some version of the claim of explanatory primacy
b. A theory of virtue

My aim in the remainder of this essay is to explore some of the difficulties of developing (b) in a way that does not compromise the distinctive character of an ethics of virtue.

8

The most familiar versions of (b) are theories of an Aristotelian kind.[10] An Aristotelian ethics of virtue will look something like this:

(1) *The claim of explanatory primacy* Right and proper conduct is con-
    duct that is contrary to no virtue (does not exemplify a vice).
    Good conduct is conduct that displays a virtue. Wrong or improper
    conduct is conduct that is contrary to some virtue (or exemplifies a
    vice).
(2) *The theory of virtue* Virtues are (a subset of the) human excel-
    lences, that is, those traits that enable one to live a characteristically
    human life, or to live in accordance with one's nature as a human
    being.

I shall not pause to consider the content of (2). It is, of course, the merest gesture toward a certain type of naturalism. What interests me at this point is the contrast with another theory in which (2) is replaced with (2'):

(1)   As before
(2') A virtue is a human trait the possession of which tends to promote human happiness more than the possession of alternative traits.

As with (2), this formulation is oversimplified. The view it oversimplifies is often called *character utilitarianism*.[11] This theory has the same structure as the Aristotelian one. The only difference comes from the second component. Is it too an ethics of virtue?

9

But if character utilitarianism is an ethics of virtue, we have not succeeded in identifying an ethics of a third kind. To see this, recall my earlier suggestion that the three central concepts of moral philosophy correspond to the three distinct types of theory that take one of these as basic: ethics of requirement, ethics of consequences, and ethics of virtue or character. Plainly, character utilitarianism belongs in the second category.[12] Even though character utilitarianism differs from its cousins in not taking the consequences of actions as the direct standard of appraisal for those actions – and hence is not consequentialist in Rawls's sense[13] – the value of the outcome of possessing and exercising certain traits is the ultimate standard of all other value. It shares with act utilitarianism the idea that the most fundamental notion is that of a good consequence or state of affairs, namely, human happiness. For these reasons, it seems better to call this general class of theories *ethics of outcome*.

In these terms the problem will be to see how to avoid classifying ethics of virtue as a species of ethics of outcome. For will not the ultimate standard of appraisal on Aristotelian theories be the idea of living properly as a human being, that is, flourishing, from which the value of virtue is derived?

The three types of theories are distinguished by what they take the fundamental moral facts to be: facts about what we are required to do, about the intrinsic or ultimate value of possible outcomes, or about people's desires, ends, and dispositions. An ethics of virtue, at least of the Aristotelian kind I have considered, will have a theory that explains the significance of various constituents of character by reference to certain necessities and desiderata of human life, in which case the basic moral facts would be facts about what is constitutively and instrumentally needed for that way of life, facts, in short, about flourishing.

The problem, then, appears to be this: any ethics of virtue that lacks a theory of virtue will be nonexplanatory,[14] but any ethics of virtue that has such a theory will collapse into an ethics of outcome. If that is so, then Rawls's classification has not been seriously challenged.

The independence of an ethics of virtue as a type of theory distinct from character utilitarianism and other ethics of outcome must depend on the special character of its theory of good. I shall consider two proposed accounts of this special character. On the first explanation, what distinguishes the Aristotelian view from character utilitarianism is its conception of virtues as constitutive of, not merely instrumental to, flourishing. This difference is conspicuous, but on the second account the difference is deeper. It is not merely that an ethics of virtue employs a different theory of what is ultimately good from that of character utilitarianism; it is that an ethics of virtue does not have that kind of theory of good at all.

10

On the first account, what distinguishes an ethics of virtue from character utilitarianism is that it takes human excellence to be at least partially constitutive of flourishing, not just instrumental. Now if there were other constituents of flourishing, it would be arbitrary to make the theory the namesake of virtue. (It should then be called an ethics of virtue plus whatever else constitutes flourishing.) Thus virtue must be construed as the sole or somehow primary constituent of flourishing, as it was by Socrates. The resultant theory construes the basic moral facts to be facts about virtue.

Here the proposed contrast turns on the theory of value rather than on the claim of explanatory primacy. As I have construed it so far, the claim of explanatory primacy asserts the primacy of virtue over action appraisal. The theory as a whole must also establish the primacy of virtue over other values. On character utilitarianism, virtues are so identified because of their relation to independent values such as happiness. According to the first account, then, an ethics of virtue must imply, in all of its components, that human excellence is the sole or at least primary constituent of what is intrinsically valuable.

11

This is an appealing account of the difference. And such a view is naturally called an ethics of virtue. Nevertheless, I doubt that this account succeeds in identifying a theory of the third kind, that is, of a kind that contrasts with both an ethics of requirement and an ethics of outcome.

Character utilitarianism is disqualified as an ethics of virtue because the facts it takes to be morally basic are not facts about virtue. However, it is not enough just to meet this qualification. For consider a restricted version of what Rawls calls perfectionism, which enjoins us to promote the development and exercise of virtue, these being intrinsically good.[15] This view meets the above qualifications, but if it is an ethics of virtue, it is so only in the way in which utilitarianism is an ethics of happiness or welfare. What fills in the blank in "an ethics of ———" merely indicates the kinds of intrinsically valuable facts or states of affairs that are taken as basic. Different terms yield different versions of ethics of outcome.

Thus if the view I have been investigating is an ethics of virtue because it takes virtue as the ultimate value, then so is perfectionism, which is an ethics of outcome. To be sure, perfectionism differs from what I have been calling an ethics of virtue in its rejection of the claim of explanatory primacy. And so it might be suggested that both an "areteic" theory of value and an "areteic" theory of right are necessary and sufficient for an ethics of virtue. According to this suggestion, an ethics of virtue stands to perfectionism as character utilitarianism stands to act utilitarianism: each pair has the same theory of good but a different theory of right.

To disqualify perfectionism as an ethics of virtue because it does not hold the claim of explanatory primacy is superficial. For unlike character utilitarianism, which in its theory of virtue goes against the grain of the primacy of virtue, the perfectionist theory of right and theory of good both hold virtue supreme. Taken together, they enjoin the fullest realization of virtue in character and action. A consequentialist theory of right is only a schema without a theory of good. When that theory is areteic, so is the theory of right. Questions of classification are, of course, relative to purpose. But for the reasons just mentioned, the kinship of perfectionism and Aristotelianism (as conceived on the first account) seems to me much closer than the relationship of character utilitarianism to either.

12

Unlike perfectionism, of course, an ethics of virtue as so far conceived is not consequentialist (in the prevalent narrow sense). But nor, as we have seen, is character utilitarianism. Consequentialist theories in the narrower sense belong to a wider class of theories that share a certain scheme of value according to which the ultimate standard of appraisal is provided by states of affairs or outcomes deemed to be intrinsically good or desirable on their own. I have been calling this wider class of theories ethics of outcome, which are characterized neither by their theories of right (which may or may not be consequentialist) nor by the specific content of their theories of good (which may range from pleasure to excellence of character) but by their appeal to this kind of scheme.

The first account of an ethics of virtue makes it a kind of ethics of outcome that is like perfectionism in its appraisal of outcomes but like character utilitarianism in the form of its conception of right conduct. I now turn to the second account, which holds that an ethics of virtue is not an ethics of outcome at all.

13

We may depict the appraisal of conduct on an (Aristotelian) ethics of virtue with the following schema:

1. Living a characteristically human life (functioning well as a human being) requires possessing and exemplifying certain traits, T.
2. T are therefore human excellences and render their possessors to that extent good human beings.
3. Acting in way W is an accordance with T (or exemplifies or is contrary to T).
4. Therefore, W is right (good or wrong).

Here there is an appeal to several notions of good: to functioning well as a human being, to being a good human being, to being a human excellence (perhaps also to being good for one as a human being). But at no stage need there be an essential appeal to the idea of a valuable state of affairs or outcome from which the moral significance of everything (or anything) else derives.

To be sure, a concern for outcomes will be internal to certain virtues. For instance, the benevolent person will be concerned that others fare well. But the moral significance of this concern stems from the fact that it is part of a virtue, not from the fact that misery and well-being are intrinsically or ultimately bad and good respectively. To put it another way, it will follow from an ethics of virtue that virtuous people care about certain things (and outcomes) for their own sakes (as final ends in themselves). There is no further commitment, however, to the idea that these concerns are virtuous ones because their objects are inherently valuable or desirable for their own sakes.[16]

Nor, more generally, is there a foundational role for the idea that living a characteristic human life is intrinsically good. Perhaps it will follow from the theory that the virtuous person *will* desire to live such a life for its own sake, and in that sense such a life can be said to be desirable for its own sake (the virtuous person being the standard), but that will be because such a desire is part of human excellence, rather than the other way around. That appraisal is made from the standpoint of virtue and is not its basis.

It may be useful to compare a theory of excellence for a nonhuman animal. The judgment that a lack of attention to her cubs is an imperfection in a mother tiger (though not in the father) is based upon a notion of a good specimen of tiger. This idea in turn depends upon what is normal for or characteristic of tigers. None of these judgments is mediated by any notion of the value of a tiger's living a life characteristic of its species. On an ethics of virtue, the same goes for people. The specific excellences will be different, of course. Moreover, for us but not for tigers there may be a point to a distinction between virtues and other excellences.

What is liable to be confusing on this account is that faring well, for example, plays a double role in this view, first in the theory of virtue, where virtues are identified in part by their contribution to a characteristic human life, and second in the theory of good, where living such a life may be among the final ends of morally admirable individuals. The distinctive feature of an ethics of virtue on the second account is that the evaluation of such a life as a final end is derivative from, rather than foundational to, the theory of virtue. On the first account, the theory of virtue is dependent on a theory of the ultimate good. On the second account, the theory of ultimate good is dependent on the theory of virtue.[17] (Hence, the fact that virtues are identified as such by their "instrumental" properties does not make them of instrumental value.)

Whatever one may think of the prospects for an ethics of virtue, this last point seems to me to be of some importance for moral philosophy. For it shows how one can assert a systematic connection between virtues and other goods without undermining the autonomy of virtue. In an outcome ethics that recognizes these goods, it is notoriously difficult to explain satisfactorily why they should not be of paramount moral concern (at least ideally), that is, how there can properly be restrictions on consequentialist reasoning. On an outcome ethics, such restrictions can never seem fully enlightened. (Hence the appearance of paradox or irrationality in "indirect" forms of consequentialism.) On an ethics of virtue, however, there is not even the appearance of a problem. For the value of virtue is not said to come from the value of anything else at all. Although it is a teleological view, an ethics of virtue can acknowledge "deontological" reasons without paradox, because it is not an ethics of outcome.[18]

In summary, on the first account, an ethics of virtue is a species of ethics of outcome, distinguished from character utilitarianism by the fact that it takes virtue and its exercise to be the sole ultimate value and from perfectionism by the fact that it does not give a consequentialist definition of right action. On this view, Rawls is right in the end to think that moral theories come in two fundamental kinds, namely (in my terminology) ethics of requirement and ethics of outcome. What his scheme overlooks is that ethics of outcome can take both a consequentialist and non-consequentialist form.

On the second account, what Rawls's scheme overlooks is more significant. Ethics of virtue contrast importantly with both ethics of outcome and ethics of requirement. The first two are teleological in that the primary notion is a notion of goodness, but they differ in the kind of theory of good that is employed. On the first account, act utilitarianism, character utilitarianism, perfectionism, and ethics of virtue are merely structural variations of an ethics of outcome. But on the second account, it is not that ethics of virtue have a different view of what outcomes are good but rather that they do not employ this notion at the foundation of the theory. The result is a teleological theory that has not received much attention or even recognition. For this reason, only the second account seems to me to identify a distinctive, third kind of moral theory.

Furthermore, only the second account yields a theory that is at bottom truly naturalistic. Admittedly, what is valuable on the first account is the natural (what belongs to human nature). But so long as the theory relies upon a primitive idea of the intrinsically or ultimately valuable outcome, the conception of value remains ungrounded. In contrast, valuable outcomes are understood on the second account by reference to the concerns of those who exemplify human nature.

14

By rejecting outcomes as the foundational standards of appraisal, ethics of virtue are, of course, allied with ethics of requirement. I complained in section 2 that the identification of teleological and consequentialist theories forces us wrongly to classify ethics of virtue as deontological. What we have now seen is that if teleological theories are those in which appraisals are guided ultimately by some notion of the good, then there are (at least) two kinds of teleological theory: those based on the notion of a good outcome and those based on the notion of good of (and for) a kind.

As I have remarked, ethics of virtue will, of course, be deontological on Rawls's negative characterization, namely, as nonconsequentialism. But if a deontological view holds more positively that "it is sometimes wrong to do what will produce the best available outcome overall,"[19] then it will not do to think of an ethics of virtue as deontological. For on this characterization, deontological views share with consequentialism the assumption that there is a coherent and acceptable way of defining "best available outcome overall" independently of the notion of right and wrong action. But an ethics of virtue is not committed to this assumption.[20]

Nor need an ethics of requirement accept this assumption. Kant, for one, would have rejected it, though he is the first to come to most people's minds when they think of "deontologists." For Kant, it may indeed turn out to be wrong to do what would in the circumstances produce the greatest overall satisfaction of desire (or to maximize any specified kind of effect), but that will not be, for Kant, a case in which acting wrongly would produce the best overall outcome. The satisfaction of desire has no value whatever when it conflicts with the moral law.

Instead of defining "deontological theory" in either of the ways just considered, it seems best simply to use it synonymously with "ethics of requirement," a useage that is in accordance with its etymology. This type of theory, as I have said, is one that takes the notion of requirement as primary to the concepts of virtue and valuable outcome. But what this means more precisely remains to be clarified. Presumably, Kant's moral philosophy, which attempts to understand moral phenomena in terms of the requirements stemming from the conditions on free agency, is to be included, as is the minimal theory of Prichard, according to which we intuitively apprehend facts about duties and obligations. One would also expect contractualism to fall under this heading. It construes moral phenomena in terms of the requirements implicit in the conditions for mutually acceptable social life. But perhaps all that these views have in common is that they are *not* teleological in either of the two ways I have identified. Is there another way? Until we understand these theories better, we cannot say.[21]

15

Despite a renewal of interest in Aristotelian ideas, ethics of virtue continue to prompt a lot of resistance. Perhaps it is worthwhile briefly to indicate why.

Many of our modern suspicions can be put in the form of a dilemma. Either the theory's pivotal account of human nature (or characteristic human life) will be morally indeterminate, or it will not be objectively well founded. At best, an objectively well-founded theory of human nature would support evaluations of the kind that we can make about tigers – that this one is a good or bad specimen, that that behavior is abnormal. These judgments might be part of a theory of *health*, but our conception of morality resists the analogy with health, the reduction of evil to defect. (This resistance has something to do, I suspect, with a conception of free will that resists all forms of naturalism.) An objective account of human nature would imply, perhaps, that a good human life must be social in character. This implication will disqualify the sociopath but not the Hell's Angel. The contrast is revealing, for we tend to regard the sociopath not as evil but as beyond the pale of morality. On the other hand, if we enrich our conception of sociality to exclude Hell's Angels, the worry is that this conception will no longer ground moral judgment but rather express it.

A related but distinct complaint concerns moral motivation. Even if we grant that we can derive determinate appraisals of conduct from an objective description of what is characteristic of the species, why should we care about those appraisals? Why should we care about living distinctively human lives rather than living like pigs or gangsters? Why is it worthwhile for us to have those particular virtues at the cost of alternative lives they preclude? There are two sorts of skepticism here. (1) Can an objective theory really establish that being a gangster is incompatible with being a good human being? (2) If it can, can it establish an intelligible connection between those appraisals and what we have reasons to do as individuals?

To answer (2) by saying "Because we are human beings" is obscure. For we are (or can be) these other things as well. "Our humanity is inescapable," it might be replied, "whereas we can choose whether or not to be a Hell's Angel."[22] The force of this reply is unclear, however, for we *can* choose whether to live a *good* (that is, characteristic) human life.

However, the point might be that we are human beings *by nature* and not these other things, and our nature determines what descriptions are essential. A good gangster is a bad human being and for that reason fails to fare well. Defective or nonvirtuous human beings are worse off for that. They are not merely bad human beings but *they* are badly off as individuals, and if they acquired virtue, they would not only be better human beings but also be better off than they would have been otherwise. Whether we are flourishing depends on who (what) we are by nature. Since we are essentially human, the description "bad human being" dominates the description "good gangster" in appraisals of well-being.

Such evaluational essentialism does not sit well with modern notions. Just as God is dead, it will be said, so the concept of human nature has ceased to be normative. We can no more recover the necessary-world view of the ancients than we can revitalize the Judeo-Christian tradition. But an ethics of virtue need not take this essentialist line. It could say instead that we care about being good human beings because or insofar as we are good human beings. Insofar as we are not, we don't (at least in the virtuous way). If we don't, then we will not flourish as human beings, though we might do very well as thieves. There is no further question to be answered here about well-being.

These seem to me to be the main worries and issues that must be faced before we can determine the prospects for an ethics of virtue. There is much to be said about what an objective account of human nature is supposed to be, as well as about the supposed disanalogies with health and about issues of motivational internalism.[23] In this section I have tried merely to indicate some of the more troublesome questions.[24]

16

I began this essay with a complaint about one of Rawls's distinctions. I shall conclude by endorsing another. In "The Independence of Moral Theory" Rawls characterizes moral theory as the systematic comparison of moral conceptions, in other words, "the study of how the basic notions of the right, the good, and moral worth may be arranged to form different moral structures" (1975, 5). He rightly emphasizes the importance of such a study quite independent of the question of which moral conception is correct. He believes that "the further advance of moral philosophy depends upon a deeper understanding of the structure of moral conceptions" and urges that "all the main conceptions in the tradition of moral philosophy must be continually renewed: we must try to strengthen their formulation by noting the criticisms that are exchanged and by incorporating in each the advances of the others, so far as this is possible. In this endeavor the aim of those most attracted to a particular view should be not to confute but to perfect" (1975, 22).

This essay is intended to be a contribution to "moral theory" in Rawls's sense. My complaint has been that Rawls's twofold classification stymies the recently renewed examination of ethics of virtue by obscuring its distinctive character. We should not be indifferent to this consequence, even if we suspect that nowadays an ethics of virtue is not something that we are going to be able to live with philosophically. For the distinctive features of this moral conception (or set of conceptions) might reveal theoretical possibilities that will help us eventually to fashion something in which we can feel more at home.

Notes

1 Rawls 1971, p. 24.
2 If maximizing is understood causally, as Rawls pretty clearly construes it, then the independence clause is implied by the definition. E cannot be said to maximize or produce G unless G is definable independently from E.
3 I agree with John Cooper: "In Aristotle's theory, human good *consists* (partly) in virtuous action, so his theory, while decidedly not teleological in the modern [consequentialist] sense, is also not deontological either" (1975, 88). See note 24 for a further discussion of Aristotle.
4 Rawls's treatment of the three main concepts of moral theory might seem infelicitous in another way. The concept of moral worth is the concept of a kind of goodness of persons. If it is derivative at all, how could this concept fail to be derived from the concept of the good, since it is an instance of that concept? The answer, I think, is that here Rawls is thinking of the concept of the good needed for consequentialist theories, the concept of a good state of affairs or outcome. See note 17.
5 At least the negative half of the primacy thesis – that wrong action is to be construed as behavior that exemplifies a vice or is contrary to a virtue – is endorsed by James Wallace: "It is a plausible thesis generally that the faulty

actions philosophers lump under the heading of 'morally wrong' are actions fully characteristic of some vice" (1978, 59).

The relation between action appraisal and character appraisal is complicated and is different for different terms of appraisal. My formulations of the primacy claim suggests that the rightness or wrongness of an action depends upon its explanation (in the person's motive or character). However, we often appraise a prospective action as the right or wrong thing to do without appraising anyone's character. We need not refer to someone's motives or character to judge that it would be wrong for her not to return a lost wallet. This observation indicates the oversimplifications of the formulations of the primacy thesis in the text. An adequate formulation would distinguish, for example, between the appraisals "*P* acted rightly or wrongly in doing *a*," and "It would be wrong (for *P*) to do *a*" or "What *P* did was the right (or wrong) thing," and it would show how all of these appraisals are implicated with standards of virtue. It might show, for example, that the standard for the right thing to do is what the morally good person would do but also that whether one acts rightly or wrongly in doing the right thing depends on one's reasons and hence on the explanation of one's behavior (or what it displays about one's character). When particular formulations of the primacy thesis are given in the text, the reader should bear these complications in mind.

A mixed view is also possible here: that priority holds in the case of some virtues and not others. I shall ignore this possibility.

6   Anscombe 1981, p. 33. I do not assert here that Anscombe is adopting an ethics of virtue. One could hold a version of the replacement thesis – that "right" and "wrong" should be replaced by "unjust," "cowardly" etc. – without holding that the latter terms can be explained by terms of character. In several forums Richard Taylor has recommended a radical version of the replacement thesis. He advanced this view in his lecture at the Conference on Virtue at the University of San Diego, February 1986. See also Taylor 1985.

7   This commitment is not peculiar to ethics of virtue. If the explanatory relation between virtue and right conduct were reversed, if, for example, a virtue were a kind of sensitivity to proper conduct within a certain sphere, then arguably the harmony thesis would follow as well. For this kind of argument, see McDowell 1979.

8   Radical replacement theories neither accept nor reject codifiability, since this question presupposes the applicability of the concepts they wish to abandon.

9   In the lecture referred to in note 6 Taylor opposes theory of this kind.

10   For the most part my discussion will be confined to roughly Aristotelian versions. See note 24 for a brief discussion of a non-Aristotelian alternative.

11   See Adams 1976. One glaring oversimplification is this. Virtues are obviously only a subset of optimizing traits. Another point is that optimizing traits cannot be determined in isolation from other traits possessed by the agent. This last point is not so easily met.

12 My concern, of course, is not with utilitarianism in particular but with consequentialism in general. There are as many different theories of this kind as there are kinds of valuable consequences that virtue(s) might foster.

13 The limits of Rawls's taxonomy is further revealed in its application to this case. Because of (1) and because character utilitarianism does not define the right as what maximizes the good, Rawls's scheme counts that view (along with all nonact forms of consequentialism) as deontological.

14 To charge intuitionism with being nonexplanatory is not an honest objection to this view, for the "objection" is precisely what intuitionism asserts: that there are no explanations of the kind we seek. This is no problem for the theory if the theory is true. So the charge begs the question. It is a "problem" only for those who wish more. So this charge (as a charge) has to be seen as an expression of one's conviction that this assertion is unreasonable. The burden will be on one who makes this charge to produce the relevant account.

15 Rawls's scheme cannot accommodate perfectionism as readily as Rawls supposes. The theory that we are to maximize excellence (where virtues are understood as human excellences) is clearly a teleological view. But it is not one in which the concept of moral worth is derived from the other concepts of the good and the right. Unlike other forms of consequentialism, perfectionism cannot accept Rawls's definition of virtues as "normally effective desires to act on the basic principles of right" (1971, 436). To avoid circularity (virtue is a commitment to maximize virtue) and to yield a teleological theory, virtues must be independently defined. On the other hand, perfectionism is not a view in which the concept of virtue is derived from the good. On this view, virtue *is* the good.

16 Christine Korsgaard (1983) has pointed out the importance of the difference between the concept of the intrinsically good and the concept of what is desirable in itself. For my purposes here, however, I do not think it matters which way I put it. An ethics of outcome may be stated either way. On the second account, an ethics of virtue has no use for the former and explains the latter by appeal to the desires of the virtuous person.

17 This constitutes my reply to a problem posed at the end of section 9 above. Insofar as virtues must in the end be characterized by their contribution to the good for human beings, that notion of the good will be primary relative to virtue. But there would still be a point to thinking of the theory under consideration as an ethics of virtue, since virtue remains basic relative to concepts of right and a good state of affairs. In the classification to which I refer at the beginning, I suspect that Rawls understands the concept of the good in that context as what is ultimately worth choosing, aiming at, seeking – that is, in effect, as the finally good outcome. So understood, on the theory I am trying to describe, virtue is prior to *that* notion, and so the priority claim is maintained. See note 4.

18 For more on deontological reasons, see the next section. My discussion here is obviously influenced by the work of Philippa Foot (1985). Foot urges that

the basic feature of consequentialism is that it employs the idea of "the best overall state of affairs." While I know of no work in which she characterizes the distinctive features of ethics of virtue as I suggest here, this characterization fits well with the writings I have seen.

19   Scheffler 1982, p. 2. This is his initial characterization of "standard deontological views." He goes on to say, "In other words, these views incorporate what I shall call 'agent-centred restrictions': restrictions on action which have the effect of denying that there is any non-agent-relative principle for ranking overall states of affairs from best to worst such that it is always permissible to produce the best available state of affairs so characterized." What follows "in other words" is not equivalent to what precedes it. An ethics of virtue will be deontological in the former sense but not in the latter.

20   See once again Foot 1985.

21   It follows from my discussion that one cannot tell whether a theory belongs to one of these types by consulting the content of its requirements or proscriptions. Conceivably, a particular version of an ethics of virtue may conclude that there is but a single virtue, the concern to produce the greatest good for the greatest number or to act only on maxims that could become universal laws for all rational beings. The same goes for contractualism; it could be argued that utilitarianism or Kantianism gives the content of the basic agreement. Moreover, many an ethics of outcome has argued for a role for "deontological constraints" in vouchsafing their favorite states of affairs. What makes these theories what they are is not their practical implications but their premises.

22   For this reply, see Wallace 1978, pp. 43–4.

23   Foot has recently explored these questions in an illuminating set of lectures, which remain, as far as I know, unpublished.

24   Did Aristotle have an ethics of virtue in the sense I have been after? The text intimates in several places that he did have, that since his theory does not comply with Rawls's scheme, it is a model for the third kind of theory I have been seeking. Surely my formulation of the second component of the theory is rightly named after Aristotle, but there is textual evidence that he did not countenance the first component, that is, the claim of explanatory primacy. The evidence I have in mind comes from the doctrine of the mean. That doctrine is a thesis about what a virtue is, namely, a state of character that is "a mean between two vices, one of excess and one of deficiency." The trouble arises when Aristotle goes on to say that this state is a mean "*because* it aims at the intermediate condition in feelings and action" (*Nicomachean Ethics* 1109a22–32). Again, "Virtue is a mean insofar as it aims at what is intermediate" (1106b28).

Such passages as these show how an intuitionist such as W. D. Ross could have found Aristotle's views so congenial. If these remarks on the mean are put together with Aristotle's remarks on uncodifiability, we get the basic intuitionist picture. If Aristotle held an ethics of virtue, one would have expected him to have said that action and desire are "intermediate," when they are, in that (because) they manifest a medial disposition. (So Aristotle is construed by Urmson, who does not consider these contrary texts.) What he said instead implies that states of character are virtues, when they are, because of the qualities of the actions and desires in which they issue.

In view of the complexity of Aristotle's texts, I do not find these passages to be conclusive. The issue must be discussed in the context of a reading of Aristotle's work as a whole. The bearing of Aristotle's treatment of *eudaimonia* in *Nicomachean Ethics*, book 1, and of the discussion of practical reason in book 6 are also important to consider. It is not clear, for instance, how to think of the aim of practical reason on an ethics of virtue. Doesn't the practically wise individual *get it right*, and can we make sense of this without reference to a standard independent of virtue? What does the individual get right, according to an ethics of virtue? (I am grateful to Gloria Rock for pressing this point in conversation.)

Meanwhile, it is somewhat disconcerting not to be able to adduce here a single clear instance of a historically important ethics of virtue in the sense I have identified. (Of course, Aquinas should be considered in this connection as well.)

My second question is this. In view of the problems engendered by the appeal to human nature, are there alternatives to Aristotelian versions of ethics of virtue? Aristotelian formulations are most familiar, but there are also hints in contemporary discussions of the possibility of a *tradition-based* theory, a theory in which the concept of tradition somehow does the work that the concept of human nature does in the Aristotelian view. (See, for example, Larmore 1987, MacIntyre 1981, and Wallace 1988. As far as I can tell, none of these writers explicitly adopts the view I sketch below.) Let me consider briefly some of the questions raised by this idea.

The idea of a tradition-based view might be expressed as follows. Morality is radically underdetermined by the abstract and universal notion of human nature employed in Aristotelian views. To be sure, nature places boundary conditions on culture, but by itself it yields no definite content for the moral life. That content can come only from particular cultures and traditions. (Although they are clearly not synonymous, I will use "culture" and "tradition" interchangeably here.) To put it another way, what is characteristically human is to be initiated into a shared way of life. Human nature must be made determinate by socialization.

So far these ideas do not suffice for an ethics of virtue. To do so, they have to be conjoined with something like the following thesis: that proper behavior (acting, feeling, and thinking properly) is acting in accordance with the virtues as these are specified and interpreted in a person's ideals that are implicit in the culture.

I am not prepared to pursue this matter further here. I shall confine myself to two observations. First, most obviously, culture-based and nature-based views need not be exclusive. Nature might determine the sorts of things that are virtues for human beings, while culture determines the specific content. This conception would allow for cultural variation within a general nature-based ideal of the human being. (See Hampshire 1983.)

The second observation is this. It may be illuminating to subsume ethics of virtue, in either a culture-based or a nature-based version, under "self-realization" ethics. That is to say, acting properly is acting in accordance with those traits that express or realize one's self, nature, or identity. Whether one is faring well depends, as I said, upon what one is. Nature-based and tradition-based views can be seen at the extremes as giving different answers to the question of what is central to human identity. On a nature-based view, one's identity is cast by one's "species-being," so to speak, whereas on the tradition-based version, the self is more particular to its culture. As I just suggested, however, this is a false opposition on the sensible view that human nature is bound up with culture. If human nature is to live in and in accordance with a tradition, then tradition-based ethics of virtue is a form of nature-based ethics of virtue.

References

Adams, R. M. 1976. "Motive Utilitarianism." *Journal of Philosophy* 73: 467–81.

Anscombe, G. E. M. 1981. "Modern Moral Philosophy." In *The Collected Philosophical Papers of G. E. M. Anscombe* (vol. 3). Minneapolis, MN: University of Minnesota Press.

Cooper, John. 1975. *Reason and Human Good*. Cambridge, MA: Harvard University Press.

Foot, Philippa. 1985. "Utilitarianism and the Virtues." *Mind* 94: 196–209.

Hampshire, Stuart. 1983. "Two Theories of Morality." In *Morality and Conflict*. Cambridge, MA: Harvard University Press.

Korsgaard, Christine. 1983. "Two Distinctions in Goodness." *Philosophical Review* 91: 169–95.

Larmore, Charles. 1987. *Patterns of Moral Complexity*. Cambridge: Cambridge University Press.

MacIntyre, Alasdair. 1981. *After Virtue*. Notre Dame, IN: Notre Dame University Press.

McDowell, John. 1978. "Virtue and Reason." *Monist* 62: 331–50 (also in this volume, pp. 105–20).

Rawls, John. 1971. *A Theory of Justice*. Cambridge, MA: Harvard University Press.

Scheffler, Samuel. 1982. *The Rejection of Consequentialism*. Oxford: Oxford University Press.

Taylor, Richard. 1985. *Ethics, Faith, and Reason*. Englewood Cliffs, NJ: Prentice-Hall.

Wallace, James. 1978. *Virtues and Vices*. Ithaca, NY: Cornell University Press.

——. 1988. *Moral Relevance and Moral Conflict*. Ithaca, NY: Cornell University Press.

Index